Turn Your
New Year's Resolution
into a
Personal Revolution:

How to Make a Resolution
and Stick to It!

Dr. Carol Stockall MD

Copyright © 2019 Carol Stockall
www.CarolStockall.com
ISBN: 9781689033152

DEDICATION

This book is dedicated to anyone who wants to make a New Year's Resolution, and this time, wants to stick to it! To anyone who has tried before and failed, my hope is that this book will give you the inspiration and instructions to succeed. Keep reading. Keep trying. Never give up.

ACKNOWLEDGMENTS

I give great thanks to the many people in my life who have helped me make resolutions and achieve my goals. I am grateful to the people who have inspired me with their success and shared the lessons of their failures. Your wisdom is contagious. You have taught me to dream big, set goals and start small. You continue to inspire me to reach higher and higher. Most of all you have inspired me to keep moving forward and never give up. Thank you!

ABOUT THE AUTHOR

People often search for solutions during times of suffering. Carol has firsthand experience seeking solutions for the suffering of her patients, her clients and herself. Hope is always her first step in healing suffering. Hope helps you begin again, dream for a different tomorrow and start taking action today.

Carol Stockall is a caregiver who has worn many hats. She began as a candy-striper, and later became a nurse, doctor, coach and counselor. A lifelong learner, Carol has a host of academic and professional letters behind her name including; BA, RN, MD, FRCPC, ACC, MC, and CCC. With decades of professional health care experience combined with a lifetime of personal experience Carol has earned a "PhD in life" that only comes with experience.

Today Carol's most known for her work coaching and counseling caregivers. She is a professional coach, certified by Erickson Coaching International, the International Coach Federation and the Physician Coaching Institute. Carol holds a post-degree diploma in Interprofessional Mental Health and a Master's degree in Counseling. Her thesis work was focused on burnout with a special interest in mindfulness to build balance and restore resilience.

Carol is dedicated to helping people achieve their goals and live their best life. Get Carol's **FREE WEEKLY PLANNER** – MAKE YOUR RESOLUTION A REALITY to help you track your resolve and keep your resolution, download it now at:

http://carolstockall.com/make-your-resolution-a-reality

The most conscientious caregivers often make caring for someone else a priority while they sacrifice their own self-care. It's easy for the life goals of the caregiver to get lost along the way. Carol helps caregivers fulfill their own goals while making life-balance and self-care a priority. Carol offers coaching, counseling and a variety of resources for caregivers seeking self-fulfillment.

For a **FREE COACHING SESSION** – MAKE YOUR RESOLUTION A REALITY contact Carol now at:

http://carolstockall.com/complimentary-coaching-session.

To connect with Carol, visit her at www.CarolStockall.com.

TABLE OF CONTENTS

PART ONE: THE NEW YEAR'S RESOLUTION 1

NEW YEAR'S RESOLUTIONS 1
The facts 1
What is a resolution? 1
HISTORY OF NEW YEAR'S RESOLUTIONS 3
BENEFITS OF NEW YEAR'S RESOLUTIONS 5
PITFALLS OF NEW YEAR'S RESOLUTIONS 7
STATS ON NEW YEAR'S RESOLUTIONS 9
WHY RESOLUTIONS FAIL 9
COMMON TYPES OF NEW YEAR'S RESOLUTIONS 11
TRENDS IN NEW YEAR'S RESOLUTIONS 13

PART TWO: THE RESOLUTION REVOLUTION 15

GOALS VS. TRADITIONAL RESOLUTIONS 15
THE POWER OF SMART GOALS 17
Dream the impossible dream 19
Turn resolutions into SMART goals 19
CHOOSING YOUR NEW YEAR'S RESOLUTION 21
Choose something you really want to change 23
Your focus matters 23
Brainstorming sessions 23
GOAL SETTING TIPS 25
Set specific goals with deadlines 25
Break down big goals into smaller goals 27
Goal setting tips checklist.. 27
Create life goals 29
Write out your goals in detail... 29
TRACKING YOUR SUCCESS 31
Create a new habit first 31
Avoiding distractions 33

EXPECT AND PREPARE FOR SETBACKS......................35
MAKE DAILY PROGRESS 37
MAKE YOURSELF ACCOUNTABLE 39
What is accountability?..39
Understanding the personal accountability.....................39
Self-empowerment..41
Personal accountability and integrity 41
Accountability in the workplace 43
Being accountable 45
Get an accountability partner...45
What is an accountability partner?...................................45
How to find your accountability partner..........................47
Accountability meetings 49
BENEFITS OF AN ACCOUNTABILITY PLAN 51
PART THREE: STICKING TO YOUR GOALS.................53
MAKE AN ACTION PLAN...53
Create a plan of action and stick to it. 53
STICKING WITH IT 57
Grit...57
Grace..57
Affirmations..57
Visualization..59
Consequences of giving into temptation..........................59
Forums and groups..59
Take a challenge 61
Bitesize your goal 61
Book a day off 63
Surround yourself with successful people.........................63
Reminders 65
Planning...67
Believe in yourself...67
Motivational Quotes..69
Ask for help 69

EXAMPLES OF ACTIONABLE STEPS **71**
Actionable steps for losing weight................................. 71
Actionable steps for exercising more.............................. 71
Actionable steps for quitting smoking........................... 73
Actionable steps for writers 73
SETTING MILESTONES...**75**
CREATE MONTHLY GOALS...**77**
SAMPLES OF GOALS **79**
Professional goals relating to career............................. 79
Personal finances 79
Business finances 79
Goals related to improving your skills.......................... 79
Health and fitness related goals 81
Dating and relationship goals...................................... 81
Family related goals 83
Travel and dream related goals 83
CONCLUSION **85**
ABOUT THE AUTHOR **87**

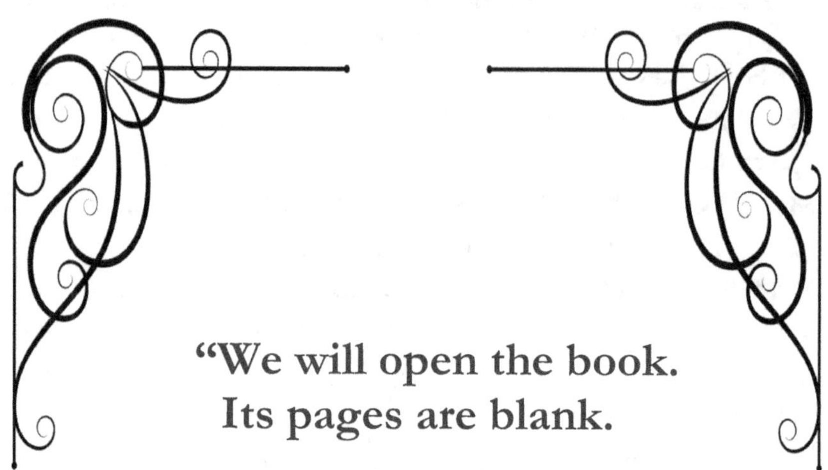

"We will open the book.
Its pages are blank.

We are going to put words
on them ourselves.

The book is called
Opportunity

and its first chapter is
New Year's Day."

~ Edith Lovejoy Pierce

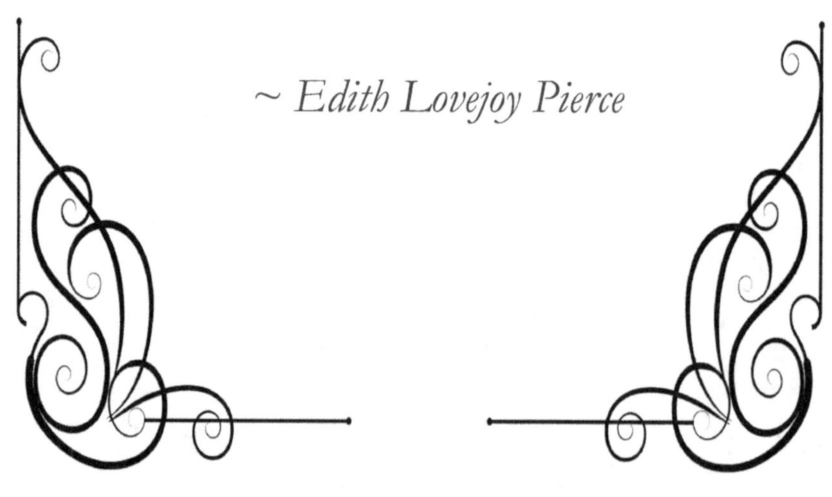

PART ONE:
THE NEW YEAR'S RESOLUTION

NEW YEAR'S RESOLUTIONS

The facts

It's easy for anyone to make a New Year's Resolution.

It's sad that many people make them knowing full well that they won't achieve them. For many people it has almost become a habit to make unattainable or unmotivated resolutions. Maybe you've been guilty of this yourself?

This is your year to change all of that! Instead of another year of resolutions quickly tossed away you can choose to make this the year you succeed!

This book is full of steps with inspiration and instructions to help you succeed. When you are done reading, you will know why people fail their resolutions, and what you can do to make sure your resolutions stick. These simple steps will allow you to set specific and reachable resolutions. You will end up with a plan of action that leaves you no choice but to succeed.

So out with the old and in with the new. Make this year the year you make a resolution and stick to it.

Enjoy the new You!

What is a resolution?

A resolution is making a promise to yourself. You promise to do something different, avoid bad habits, or to strive for a certain goal. While a resolution can be made at any time of the year the majority of people make resolutions on the 1st day of the New Year.

People want to welcome the New Year with positive change. This book will help you open new doors of possibility to cross the threshold of positive change.

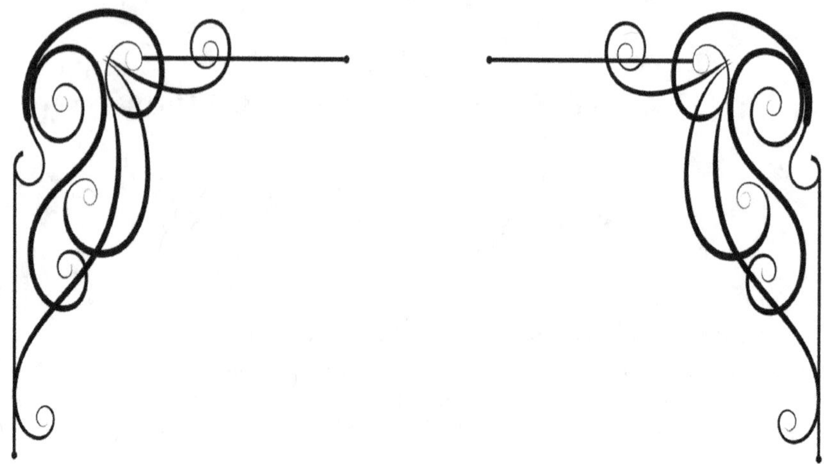

"Be at war with your vices, at
peace with your neighbors,
and let every new year find you
a better man."

~ *Benjamin Franklin*

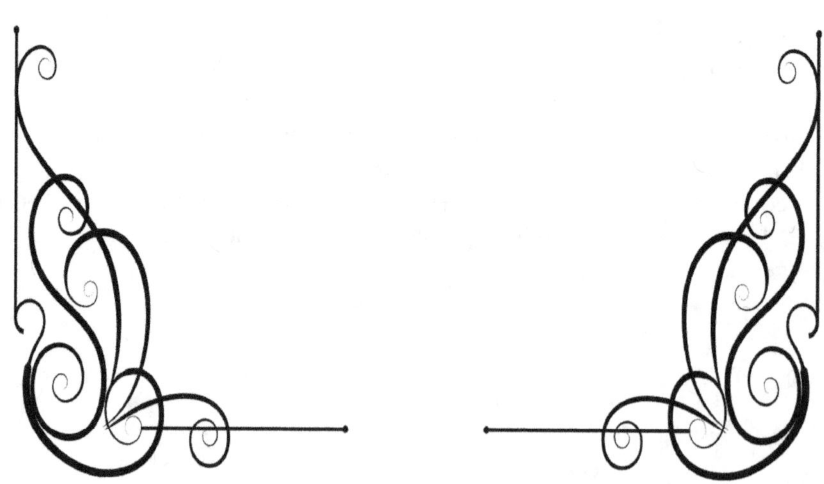

HISTORY OF NEW YEAR'S RESOLUTIONS

The actual celebration of the New Year can be traced back to pre-Christian times. The Babylonians celebrated the New Year in March, and later on the Romans would change this to January. New Year's resolutions are almost as old as the tradition of celebrating the New Year itself.

The ancient Babylonians made promises to their God's at the start of each year. These promises revolved around things like returning borrowed items or paying back debts. The Romans began each year by making promises to the god Janus. Does that name sound familiar? It should - that is where the month January got its name! In the Medieval Era, knights would take what was known as a "Peacock Vow". At the end of the Christmas season they would re-affirm their commitment to chivalry. Religious events like Judaism's Rosh Hashanah and the Catholic Lent were also an inspiration for New Year's Resolutions as we know them.

American writer Jonathan Edwards, who was a New England Puritan, took to writing out memorable New Year's Resolutions. Some people say that his written resolutions were an art form and at the age of 20 he had compiled and written a list of 70 resolutions. Apparently, he reviewed these on a weekly basis.

Our history is full of ideas of committing to self-improvement. These commitments to self-improvement are what lead to the modern New Year's Resolutions. Since these resolutions are a tradition that has stood the test of time it is likely that the tradition will continue for years to come.

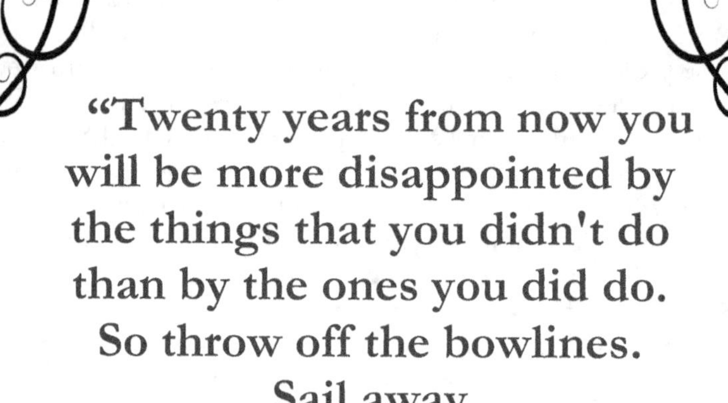

"Twenty years from now you
will be more disappointed by
the things that you didn't do
than by the ones you did do.
So throw off the bowlines.
Sail away
from the safe harbour.
Catch the trade winds
in your sails.

Explore.

Dream.

Discover."

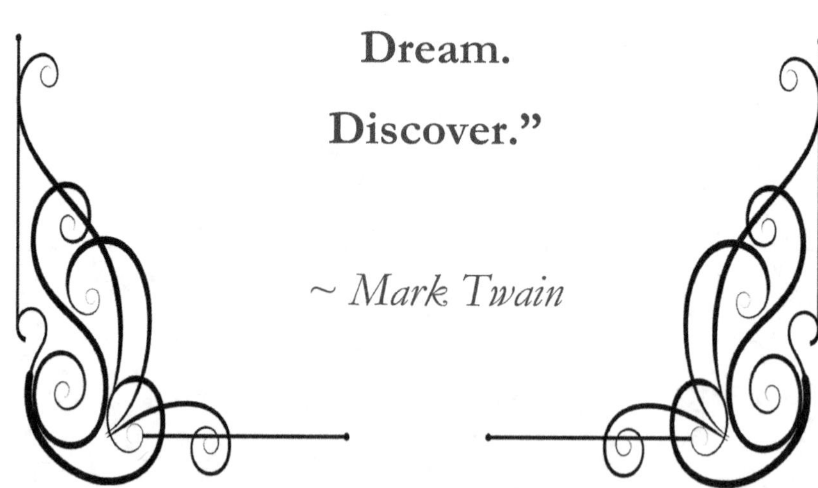

~ *Mark Twain*

BENEFITS OF NEW YEAR'S RESOLUTIONS

The biggest benefit of making a New Year's Resolution is that it can motivate you into taking action.

Of course, making a resolution isn't enough, you still need to take the required steps to achieve your goal though. The first day of a New Year is the perfect time for a fresh start. You can take a good look at your life and see what is working and what isn't and then decide what improvements you would like to make.

By making a New Year's Resolution you are taking control of your life and acknowledging that you have the power to change it. This can be a powerful step and one that can help you get out of a bad situation or to just get your life back on track. When you successfully tackle a resolution, you will find that you feel a wonderful sense of achievement at doing so. Your confidence level will soar as will your self-esteem.

If you haven't felt proud of yourself recently now is the time to sit down and come up with a powerful New Year's resolution.

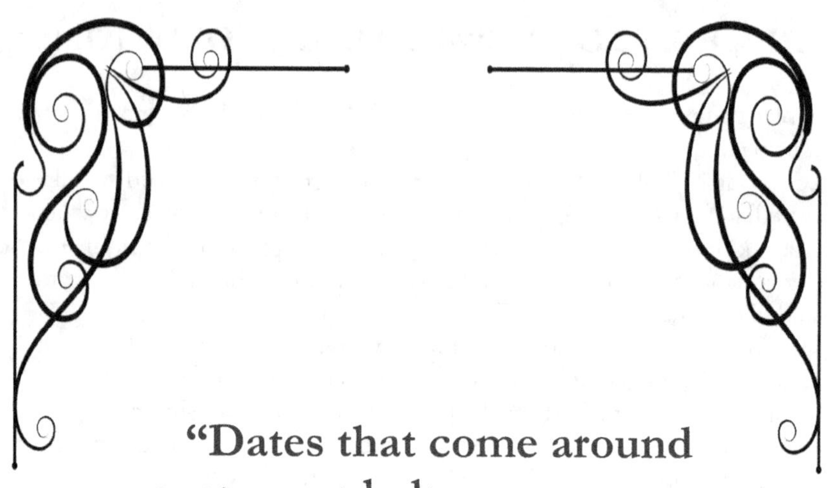

"Dates that come around
every year help us measure
progress in our lives.
One annual event,
New Year's Day,
is a time of
reflection and resolution."

~ *Joseph B. Wirthlin*

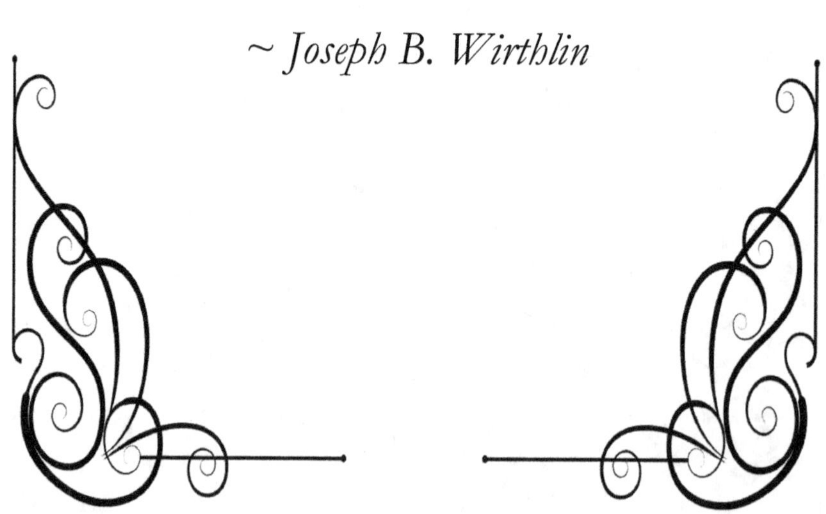

PITFALLS OF NEW YEAR'S RESOLUTIONS

While a New Year's resolution can be a powerful and motivational tool it can become a downfall for many people. This is why it is so important to set and approach your resolution correctly.

One common pitfall is beginning a resolution when your mind is not ready for it. If you are the type of person who makes the same resolution each year you need to understand why you are not achieving it.

It is very easy to make a New Year's resolution but to keep it you must follow it through with action. For example, if you are not motivated enough to lose weight don't just make a resolution to lose 10 pounds by spring. Instead take a deep look inside and explore your feelings about losing weight.

This can be an extremely difficult exercise to do. It requires being honest with yourself and this can open up some very unexpected emotions. Basically, what this boils down to, is that you need to make a New Year's resolution that is right for you.

Your resolution really has to have a powerful meaning for YOU! If you take steps because you feel pressured to do so, the end result could actually damage you as opposed to helping you. Make resolutions as promises to yourself not someone else.

If you are having trouble coming up with a definitive goal it could help to talk to a counsellor, a professional or a person you trust. This also applies if you have tried to make changes in your life and just cannot reach your goals, seeking advice could be a positive solution.

Another pitfall of New Year's resolution is that it can allow you to become extremely self-critical. If you set yourself up with an unattainable resolution, failing to reach it might make you feel worse. This is a potentially damaging downward spiral of emotions.

Remember a year is a long time and if you force yourself to stick to something, without allowing yourself to go off course, you may never achieve your goal. Do not punish yourself if you go off track. Just identify that you have done, and the reason why and then just get back on track as soon as possible. By doing this you will see much better results with your resolution.

Your mindset is going to change during the year as well and this can have an impact on your resolution. While you may begin your journey with one specific goal and with one reason in mind, all of this can change. As your journey unfolds you may discover a deeper reason for your commitment, or you may find that this was not your main focus after all.

If this does happen to you it can be a positive thing. Again, allow yourself the opportunity to shift gears and or go off course into a totally new direction.

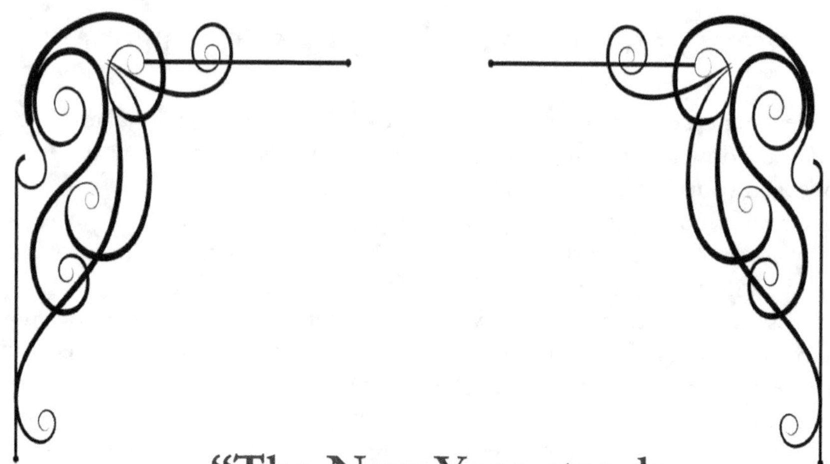

"The New Year stands
before us, like a chapter in a
book, waiting to be written.
We can help write that story by
setting goals."

~Melody Beattie

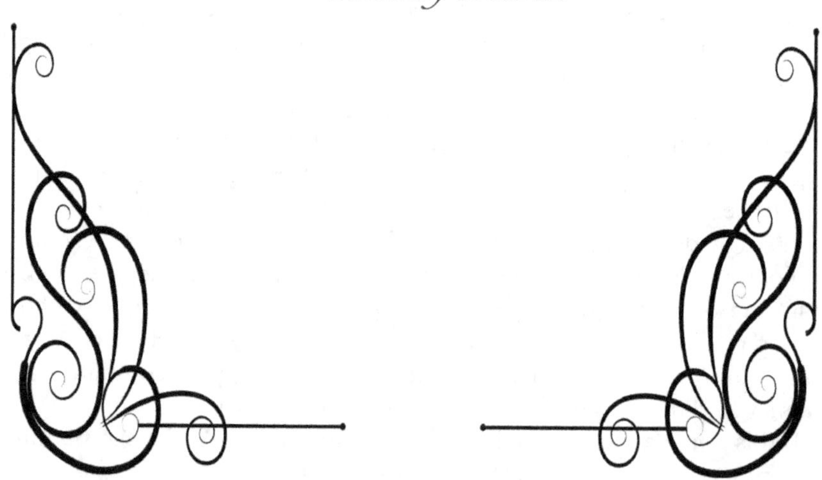

STATS ON NEW YEAR'S RESOLUTIONS

According to a variety of surveys the typical top New Year's resolutions are:
- Lose Weight
- Get Organized
- Spend Less or Save More
- Get Fit

The typical timelines and success rates
- 45% of people make yearly New Year's Resolutions
- 8% are successful and keep their New Year's Resolution
- 24% who make New Year's Resolutions never succeed
- 75% are successful throughout first week
- 72% are successful for the first two weeks
- 64% stick it out for six months
- 46% stay with it after six months

WHY RESOLUTIONS FAIL

The main reason why New Year's resolutions fail usually comes down to one of three things:
1. People make too many resolutions at one time.
2. People make impossible resolutions.
3. People make resolutions that are too vague.

The best advice for anyone starting a resolution is to make one at a time and make it simple and specific.

Don't fall into the dogma of resolutions just being a January thing. You can set a small specific goal in January, achieve it by February, and make another! I This is a good way to approach a more involved series of resolution and helps you see that it is attainable.

Other reasons for failing resolutions:
1. Lack of Willpower: The area of willpower is kind of controversial these days. Some people see it has an actual exhaustible resource that you can drain. Other's see it as just simple mind over matter.
2. "False Hope Syndrome": When your resolution is unrealistic and out of alignment with your internal view of yourself. It means you might not only fail your resolution; you might damage your self-esteem.
3. Cause and Effect: You may think that achieving your resolution will change your life or make you happier. If it doesn't you may get discouraged and revert back to your old behaviors.

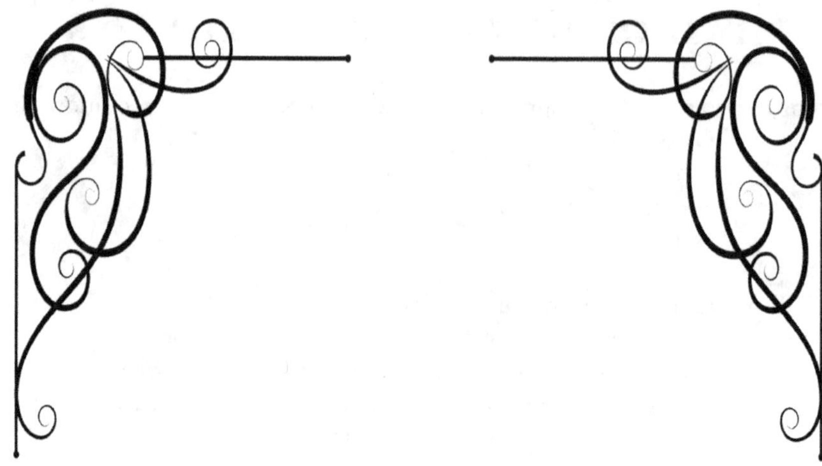

"Hope
smiles from the threshold
of the year to come."

~ Alfred Lord Tennyson

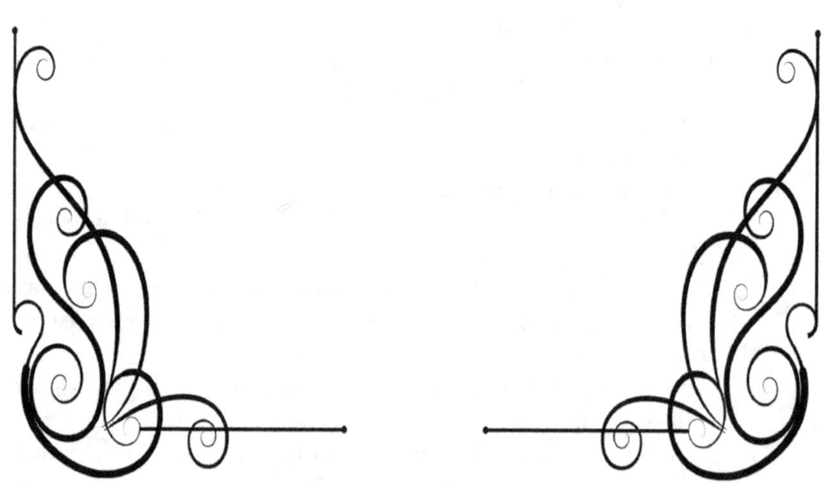

COMMON TYPES OF NEW YEAR'S RESOLUTIONS

Let's look at some common New Year's resolutions that are made by millions of people each year.

- Getting healthy: making healthy food choices, losing weight, exercise more often, to stop drinking alcohol, quit smoking, stop biting nails, to stop or get rid of any type of bad habit.
- Mental well-being: being more positive, smiling more, laughing more often and just to enjoy life and what it has to offer.
- Financial: getting out of debt, saving money, invest money.
- Career Choices: do better at work, go after that promotion, find a better job, start your own business.
- Education: get better grades, upgrade your education, learn something new for fun, learn something new to improve your career, develop good study habits, read more often.
- Self-Improvement: becoming more organized, learn to manage stress, reduce your stress, be happier, improve time management, become more independent, watch less TV, spend less time playing video games, develop a new skill.
- Go on a trip.
- Make new friends.
- Volunteer and help others out in a hospital, boys and girls club, senior home, work part time in a charity organization, help at an animal shelter.
- Spend more time with your family.
- Decide it is time to settle down.
- Try something new such as a new food or a new culture.
- Be more spiritual.
- Start a meditation practice.
- Learn to get along with people better and improve your social skills.

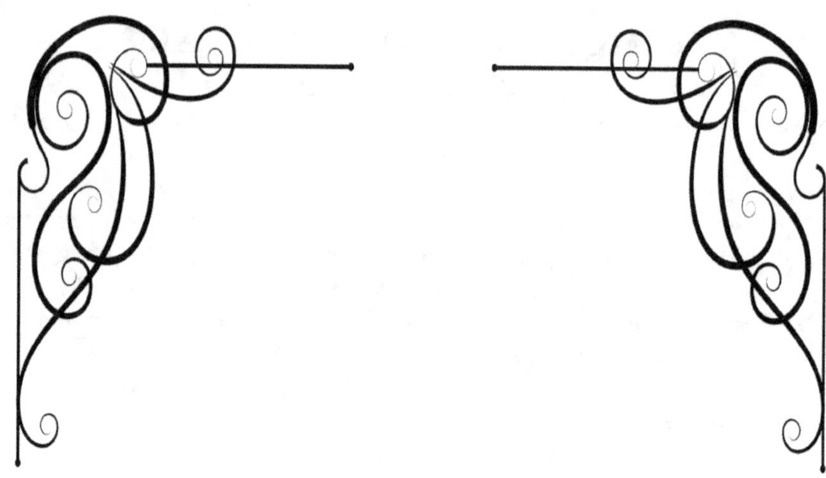

"It is with love and joy
that I create
the New Year
and
the New Me."

~ *Louise Hay*

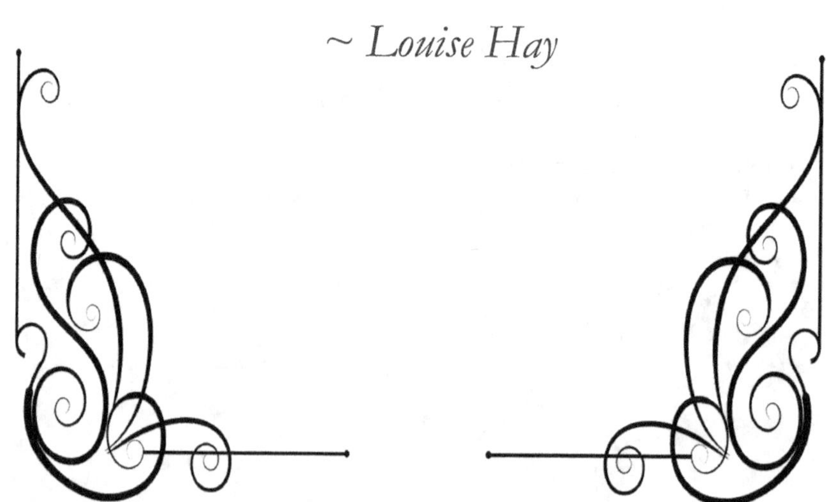

TRENDS IN NEW YEAR'S RESOLUTIONS

The trend for New Year's resolutions is that they are based on improving an aspect of your life. This can be to improve your appearance or even to renovate your home so that it is more modern.

Many people set resolutions around their home including making the time to remove all the clutter from it. It is amazing how much stuff you can accumulate over the years. This can really mount up after your children have left home and you are left with a lot of their belongings. While some things you will want to keep as memories, there will be many things that are never used and turn into a dust collector. Your resolution could be to clean this up and hold a huge garage sale. Or you may want to donate the items to a charity.

With the increase in people working online this is also a popular area for New Year's resolutions. You may want to improve your blog or website with a new theme so that it looks clean and crisp. Your goal or resolution may be to add more blog posts to your site.

Other resolutions that are related to a business include learning website design, taking a writing course or learning how to market more effectively online. Now with the popularity of mobile devices a great resolution would be to make sure that your site is mobile friendly. Otherwise you could be losing a lot of website traffic.

Learning a new skill or taking up a new hobby is much easier today because of the internet. Instead of having to pay for music lessons you can easily learn by watching YouTube videos. Want to learn art, sewing, knitting or cooking? Use online videos. They are accessible and allow you the freedom to learn at your convenience all from the comfort of your own home.

Just a few years ago none of these things would have been considered New Year's resolutions at all. Of course, the top trends for New Year's resolutions never seem to change and these are based around weight loss and exercising more.

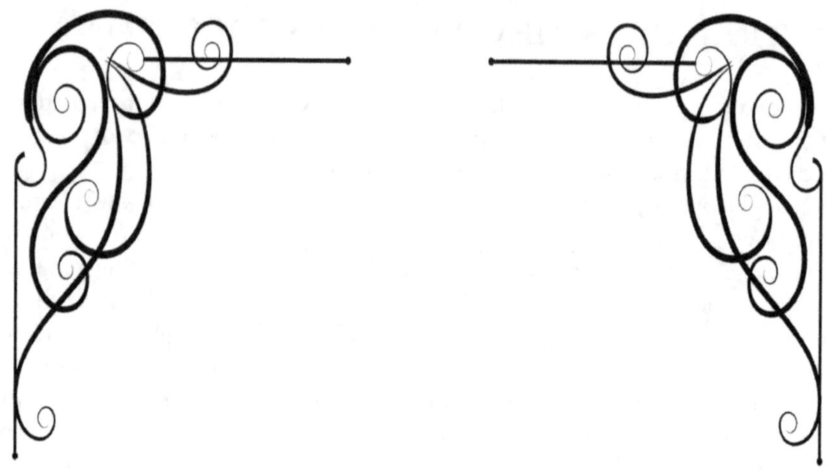

"If you want to
live a happy life,
tie it to a goal,
not to people or things."

~ *Albert Einstein*

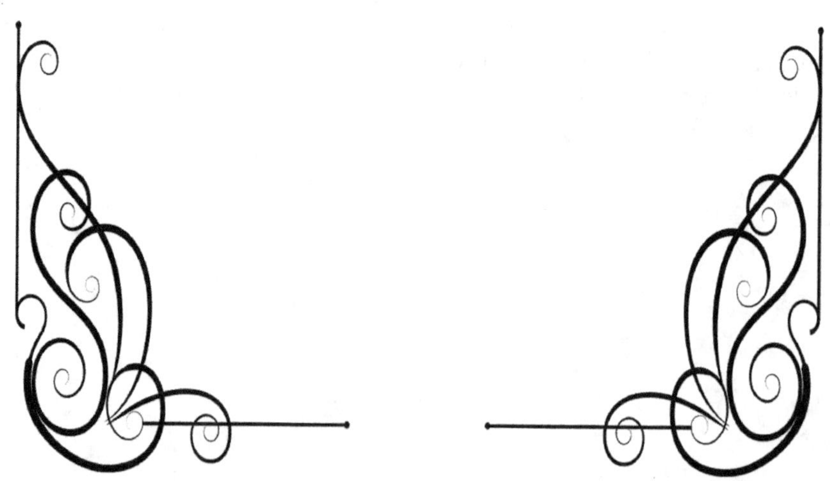

PART TWO:
THE RESOLUTION REVOLUTION

GOALS VS. TRADITIONAL RESOLUTIONS

Setting a goal is not the same thing as making a resolution.

- A typical Resolution: You want/wish/hope something to happen.
- A Goal: Something you actively work towards daily.

- A typical Resolution: A vague notion of what you want to achieve (losing weight).
- A Goal: Is specific and can be measured (losing 10 pounds)

- A typical Resolution: I'll accomplish this sometime this year (lose weight next year).
- A Goal: Has a specific time frame (lose 10 pounds in 10 weeks).

As you can see above, your typical New Year's resolution lacks the clear definition, measurability and built in accountability of a well written goal. This is why you have to set a resolution just like you would set a specific goal!

By defining your resolutions as goals, you may find that your motivation is much higher and your resolutions much more attainable.

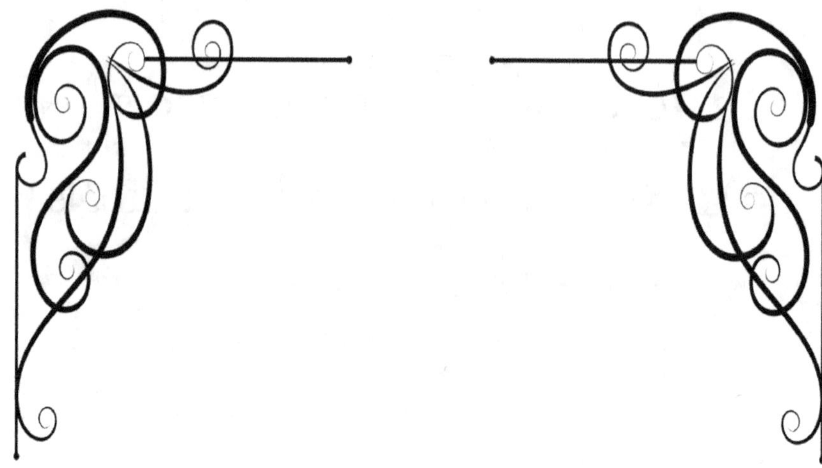

> **"A goal is a dream
> with a deadline."**

~ Napoleon Hill

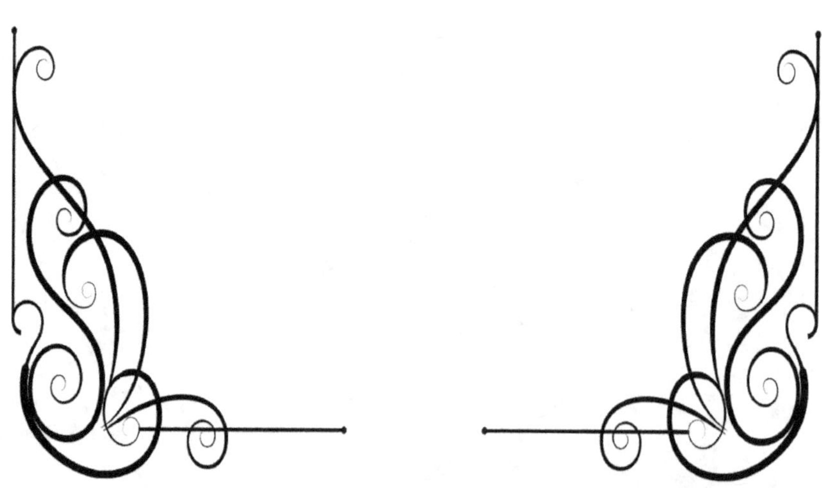

THE POWER OF SMART GOALS

When people think about goal setting, they often think of the SMART acronym:

- Specific
- Measurable
- Attainable
- Relevant
- Time based

By incorporating each of these points together you are significantly more likely to attain your goals. These points need to be explored and defined further.

Let's discuss this.

Setting a specific goal means you avoid being vague. You state clearly what your goals are with specific steps with measurable outcomes. Instead of "I want to lose weight" you say, "I want to lose ten pounds in the next 3 months."

A measurable goal helps you see things that are working for you. Then you can simply do more of what works. Continuing with the weight loss theme, the act of weighing yourself is measuring your progress. If you weigh more, you need to analyze what isn't working. If you weigh less, you can continue with what you are doing.

Attainable goals will keep success within your grasp. When your goal is within realistic reach your motivation to try harder stays with you. While you want to set attainable and achievable goals, don't make them so easy that you can reach them with your eyes shut.

Relevant goals resonate with you personally. You will be so excited by the prospect of reaching them that you maintain the motivation needed to keep going. As you begin achieving your goals, or as life changes, your goals could possibly become less relevant. This is why it is important to review them and change them as necessary.

Time based goals tie your goals to a deadline. When this happens, your sense of urgency is heightened. You won't relax on your goals because you know there is only so much time to achieve them.

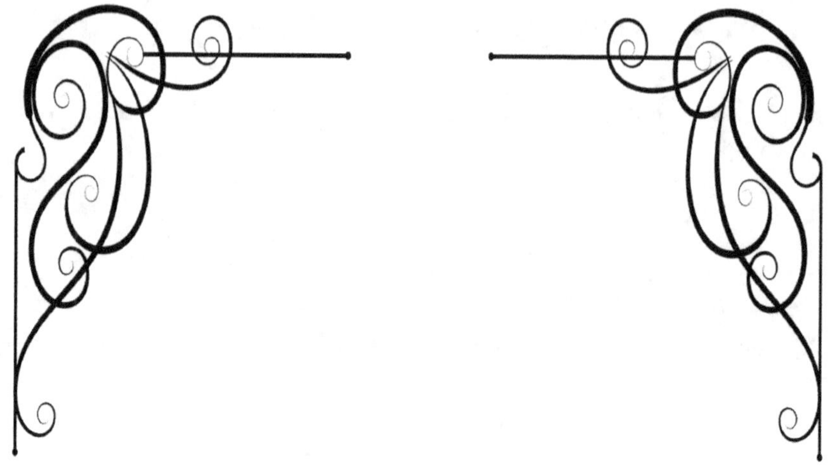

"It's kind of fun to do the impossible."

~ *Walt Disney*

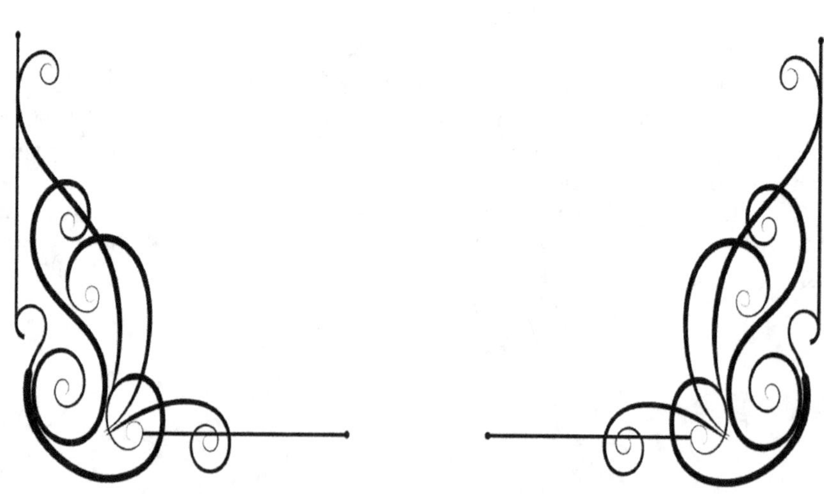

Dream the impossible dream

There is also value in setting big time, potentially unrealistic goals. While you should have SMART goals to work towards on the regular, having a larger overall dream or passion should not be discouraged. Impossible dreams can be accomplished. Dream big but start small.

Turn resolutions into SMART goals

The best way to get started with turning any New Year's resolution into a goal is to write out a list of all the things you consider to be a resolution. Once you have this in front of you it will be easy to see if some of these resolutions all have something in common. Could they be classified as one larger resolution? If they can, your goals would be as simple as completing each, one step at a time.

The worst thing about making resolutions is that you can end up with so many of them. Most people have a huge bucket type list when it comes to resolutions. If this is true for you, then you want to go through your list and prioritize by importance.

Attack the most important first.

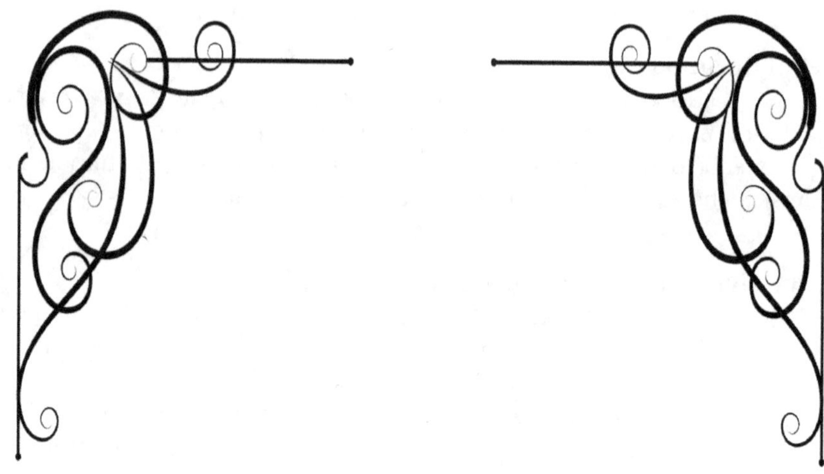

"If your dreams
don't scare you,
they aren't big enough."

~ *Lowell Lundstrum*

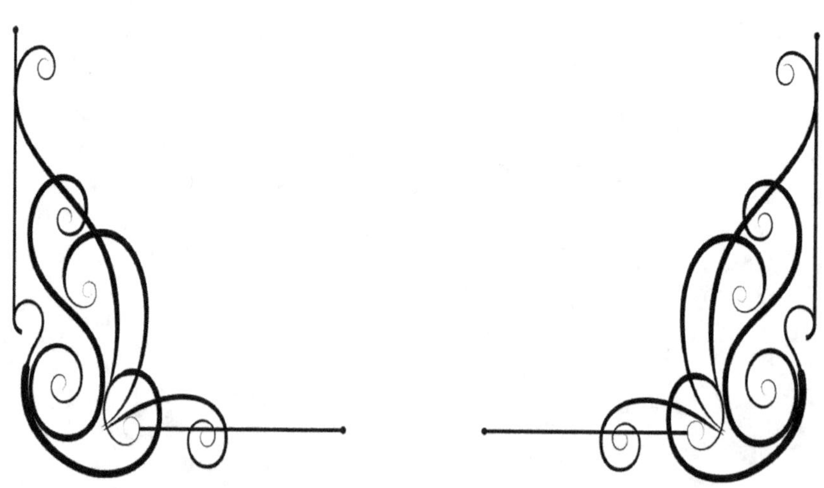

CHOOSING YOUR NEW YEAR'S RESOLUTION

Are you ready to make a New Year's resolution this year? If so, you are like many millions of people around the world that are preparing to do the same thing. Sometimes it can be hard to settle on just one resolution and this often leads people to make lots of small resolutions instead. Too many resolutions may make it difficult to focus and difficult to stay motivated.

Instead, your best option this year is to find one resolution that you want to make and then focus all your energy on attaining that one goal. This can be more difficult than it sounds. So how do you just settle on one New Year's resolution this year?

Your first step in choosing your resolution will be to start making a list of all the resolutions that you were thinking about making. Once your list is completed, you want to start examining it so that you can prioritize your resolutions. Your end goal is to have a list with your most wanted resolution sitting on top.

Quite often when you start writing out your list you may find that many of your resolutions are intertwined and can be combined into one main resolution. Each portion could be defined as its own step in the process of achieving your resolution.

Your list may contain resolutions that involve buying a new home, saving additional money and changing careers. All of these could be classified as one resolution as they are all required to achieve your end goal of buying a larger home for your family.

You would divide this resolution into smaller steps. These steps would include steps such as setting up a weekly savings plan, sending out five resumes each week or taking a course to improve your skills, so that you can apply for a new job. If you look at them from a logical viewpoint you can see how one builds upon another. They are all required in order to succeed with your resolution. So, go through your list and group items together that relate to one main goal.

Your end result may be a list that only has two or three resolutions, and this makes it much easier for you to choose one as your main focus. You need to start somewhere with your resolutions so pick the one that has the highest priority for you. This could be one that is health related or one that is related to your finances.

Once you have decided on your New Year's resolution make a point to tell your family and friends about it. Once you publicly commit to a resolution your motivation will be that much higher to actually achieve it. Public accountability is a powerful motivation for success.

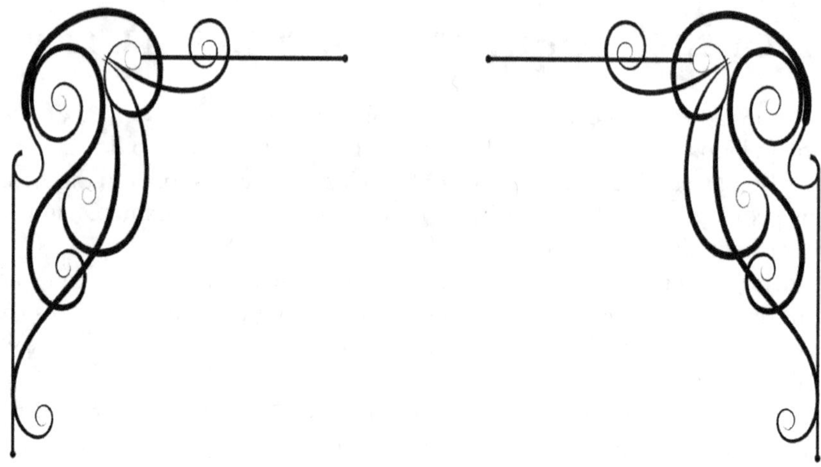

"You don't have to see the
whole staircase
to take the first step."

~ *Martin Luther King Jr.*

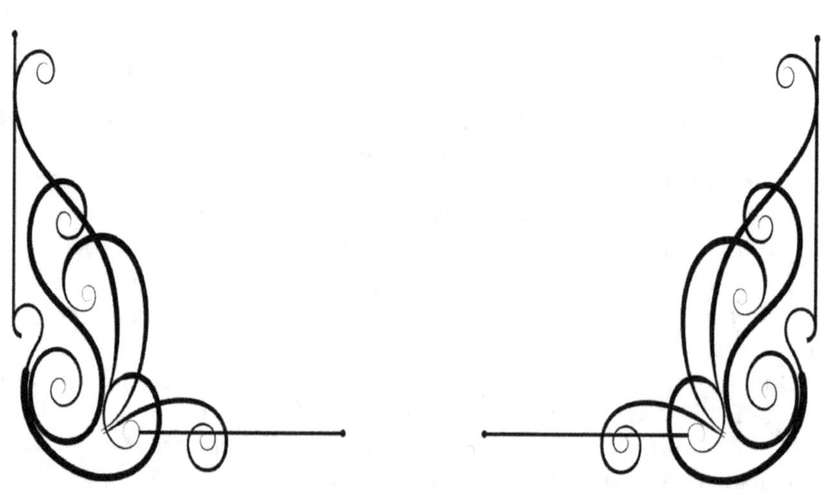

Breaking your resolution into smaller chunks will also make it easier for you to keep working on it daily. If your resolution is based around buying a new home, then work backwards and write out all the steps you need to take to make this come true. This might include going into tons of detail like knowing exactly each week or month how much money you should be saving. The more detail you include the clearer you path to your goal will be.

By outlining all the required steps your path to completing your resolution will be embedded in your mind and will help keep you motivated until you reach it.

Choose something you really want to change

Your aim here is to discover the ONE thing that you TRULY want to accomplish this year. This will become your GOAL.

Identifying just one thing can be really hard and it may take a little soul searching to find your true desire. Once you have identified it, it will be much easier for you to stay focused on just this one thing. Plus, your chances of success are greatly increased as well.

Pick one goal to focus on this year and be determined to stick with it!

Your focus matters

Most people realize that focus is important. It's easier to focus on one thing at a time. If you do have one of those 'bucket' lists narrow it down to one choice first.

There's no reason why you cannot get more accomplished during the course of the year, but just focus on one task at a time until it's complete or until you have it under control.

Brainstorming sessions

A brainstorming session can help you identify the necessary steps you need to take in order to achieve your goal. For this session you may want to use a whiteboard, a spreadsheet or good old-fashioned pen and paper.

You might find it easier to work backwards for this process. You know what your end goal is. Your goal now is to discover the steps you need to attain it. By working backwards, you can plan out steps the necessary steps.

If you love online tools then consider using a mind mapping software, there are many free ones available. Then you can easily create a mind map of where you are right now and map a path to where you want to be next month or by the end of the year. The great thing about a mind map is that you can easily add things to it as needed. Don't forget to use it to track your progress as well.

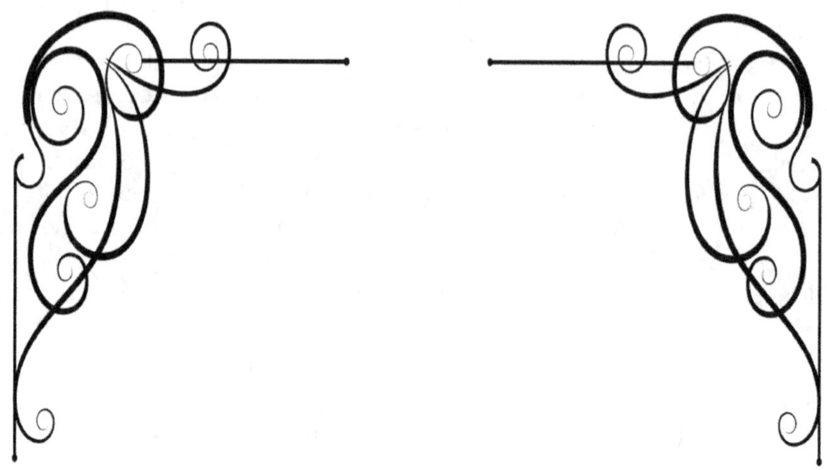

"Start
by doing what is necessary;
then do what's possible;
and suddenly you are doing
the impossible."

~ *St. Francis of Assisi*

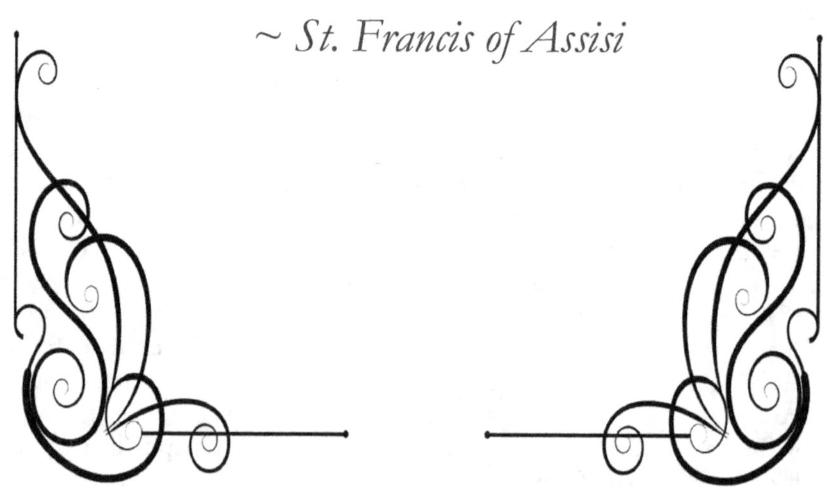

GOAL SETTING TIPS

When setting new goals, you want to create goals that really mean something to you. They must be goals where you are prepared to put your energy into them. The worst thing you can do is to make a New Year's Resolution or goal just because all your friends are making them. If you do create a resolution make sure it is something which is meaningful to you.

Have a plan of action in mind on how you are going to achieve your goal. Are you going to join a weight loss group, buy a piece of fitness equipment or throw away your lighters and ashtrays?

Remember that any goal will take time to achieve.

You must believe that you are capable of changing. If you were suddenly put into a dangerous situation you would have to adapt. What would you do if your home got damaged in a tornado? You would survive and find a way to go on. Think of achieving your goal in a similar way.

Don't view your goal as an all or nothing situation. Life happens and you will hit stumbling blocks. Take them in stride and then just get back on track. While you want to focus on your goal you do not want to make it the focal point of everything you do.

Set specific goals with deadlines
Your goal needs to be as specific as possible. This way it will be easier for you to achieve it and by setting a time frame for yourself you can stay motivated.

A specific goal is one which is really defined such as:
- I will lose 50 pounds by Dec 31st
- Compare this to a non-specific goal:
- I want to lose 50 pounds

By not setting a date you are setting yourself up for failure. You have nothing to be accountable for and no way to measure your daily or weekly success.

When it comes to setting specific goals, they need to match your expectations and your lifestyle. For example, your goal in life may be to buy a $600,000 home. This is not going to be possible if your income is only at $45,000. Your first goal should be to find ways to increase your income.

If you set unrealistic goals, you will find that you just cannot achieve them. You will end up feeling dejected and want to just give up on life in general. Instead focus on a goal that is doable and get it done.

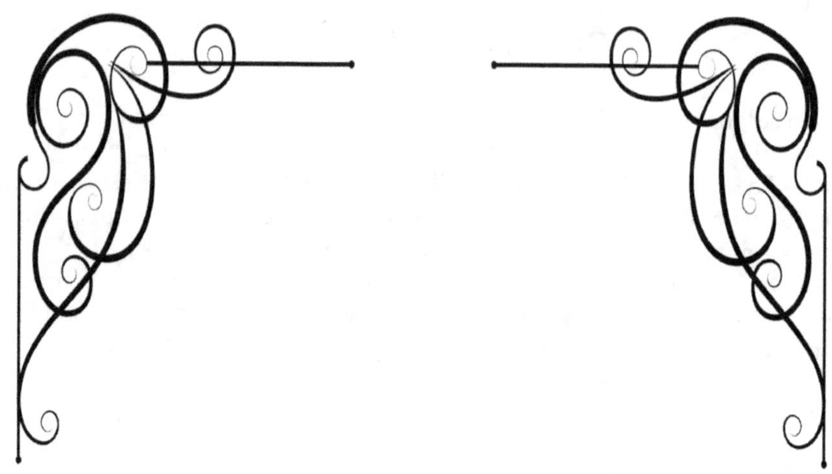

"Start where you are.

Use what you have.

Do what you can."

~ *Arthur Ashe*

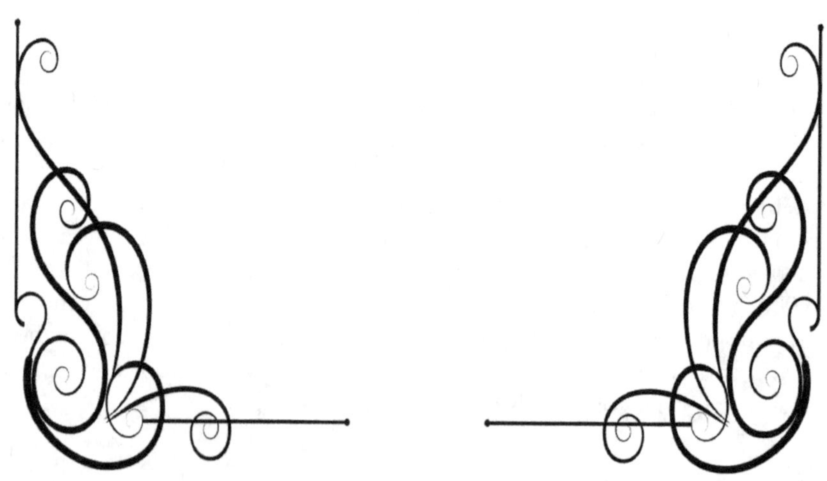

Break down big goals into smaller goals

This is where you want to look at your bigger goal such as buying a new home or losing 50 pound and creating a path to it.

Using our 50-pound goal from above you can set smaller goals such as:

- I will lose one pound per week this year
- I will lose four pounds per month

Other related smaller goals could be things like:

- giving up one can of soda each day on the weekends
- getting up 30 minutes earlier and spend the time using your treadmill

When you divide a goal into smaller chunks it immediately becomes more manageable. You won't feel as overwhelmed and you will feel as though this is something that you can actually achieve this time.

Goal setting tips checklist

A point form collection of goal setting tips

- Goals should truly mean something to you.
- Have a plan of action.
- Plot the steps towards achieving your goal.
- Break large goals up into smaller manageable goals.
- Believe in your ability.
- Goals can change, be flexible.
- Make your goals specific not vague.
- Set due dates for all the steps towards your goal
- Set realistic goals.
- Don't be afraid to dream big and have big goals as well.
- Identify and avoid behaviors that keep you from your goal.
- Use mind mapping software (or traditional brainstorming methods) to plot the steps to your goals.
- Visualize your success. Imagine what achieving your goals would mean to your life.
- Write your goals down.
- Share your goals with those important to you. They will help you along the way and hold you accountable.
- Reward yourself for achieving goals.
- Do something every day to move towards your goal.

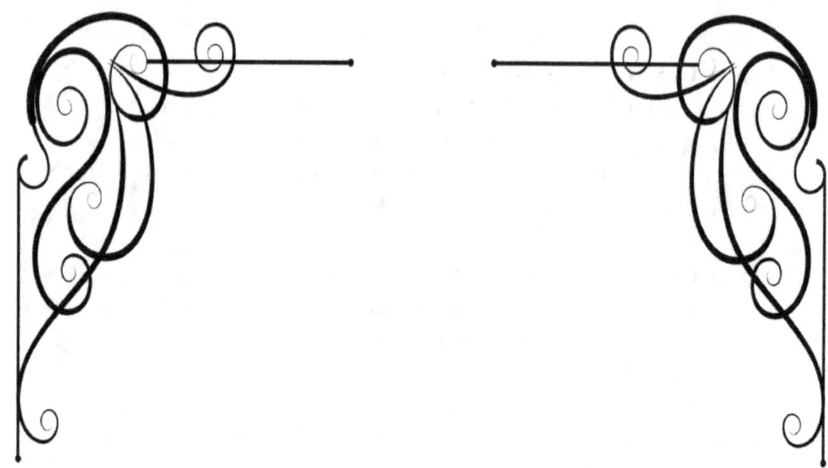

"Go after your wish.

**As soon as you start
to pursue a dream,
your life wakes up and
everything has meaning."**

~ Barbara Sher

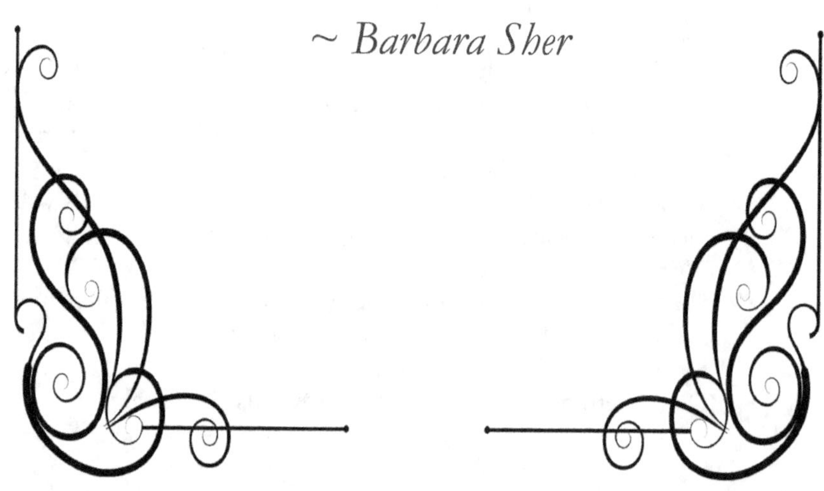

Create life goals

Many experts advocate setting individual goals for certain areas of your life. Some of the main areas recommended include:

- Family and Home Life Goals
- Financial and Career Related Goals
- Spiritual and Ethical Goals
- Physical and Health Goals
- Social and Cultural Goals
- Mental and Educational Goals

By setting a goal for each area of your life it is thought that your entire life will be more rounded. Use the above guidelines to set new goals for the coming year. You may even find that some of your goals overlap into several areas of your life, this can have a beneficial impact as you work towards them.

Write out your goals in detail

This can be a great way to really see what your goal entails and it can help you plan out how to reach your goal. Let's take the example of wanting to buy a larger home for your family.

Write out a full-blown description of how the house looks. Include the main features you want the house to have such as a three-car garage, a swimming pool, a separate entrance or nanny suite.

Then continue this by writing how the area around your home looks. Imagine you can see the mountains from your backyard, how much land do you own, what kind of trees are on your property and more.

The end result of your descriptive writing should be that you could close your eyes and picture your new home on your property, with yourself standing in the yard looking at your garden full of flowers!

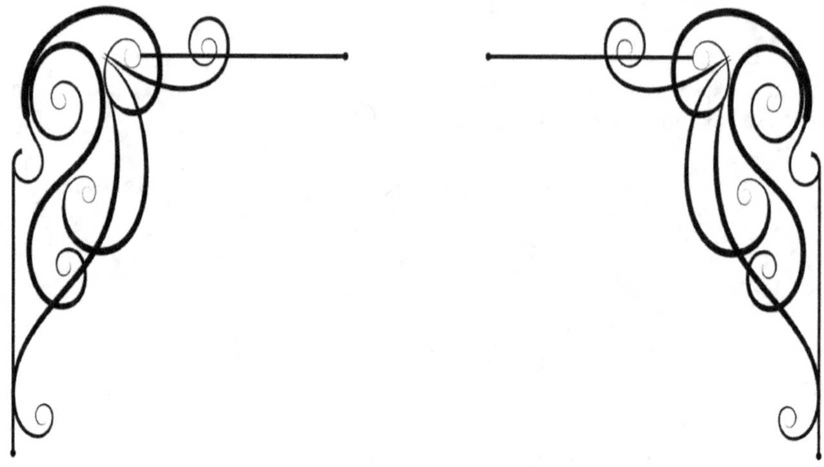

**"Success is the alignment of
positive attitude
with positive action."**

~ Carol Stockall

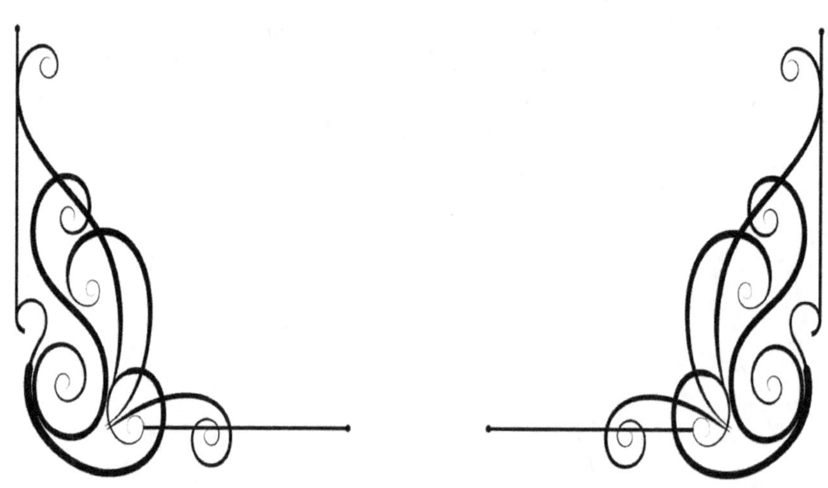

TRACKING YOUR SUCCESS

After writing out your goals you should always plan to track your success. This can be as simple as keeping a food journal and writing down each bite and lick of food you eat each day. This allows you to see if you are on track and it can expose certain areas that require more attention.

Staying with the food journal you may notice that the weekends are where you often eat more calories. It might be the time where you add in that extra beer or glass of wine or skip your exercise. Instead of not allowing yourself a treat on the weekend add it into your calorie count. This way you won't feel as though you are cheating. You won't be going over your calorie allowance either.

On the other side of the coin you may notice that you aren't eating enough calories and actually have to eat more food. If you weren't tracking your progress you wouldn't be able to identify problem areas as quickly. What you think you are doing is not always what you *are* doing!

You can track any goal that you set for yourself. If you are saving for a new home use a scheduled transaction to withdraw money to a saving account. This way you are regularly putting money into savings for this purpose only. Look at your deposit dates and make sure that money is going into your account each week or month. If not look for reasons why not.

If your goal is to save money, you may find that you have to miss a week when your rent is due or that you had an unexpected bill. Look for a way to make up the difference. Perhaps sell a service or something you no longer need. Or you might decide that you want to speed up the process by putting more money away or by taking on a part time job for a little while.

Create a new habit first

If your goal is large you can make it easier to achieve by creating lots of small habits first. Instead of trying to revamp your entire life at one time to fit a large goal, try changing small things one at a time.

Examples of small habits:

- Eat a banana at breakfast each day.
- Put five dollars into a savings account each Friday.
- Take the stairs up to your office each morning.
- Spend ten minutes exercising each day.
- Park your car at the back of the parking lot.
- Get off the bus one or two stops earlier and walk to work.
- Walk to the corner store for milk and don't drive there.
- Go to bed half an hour earlier each night.
- Do a daily act of kindness.

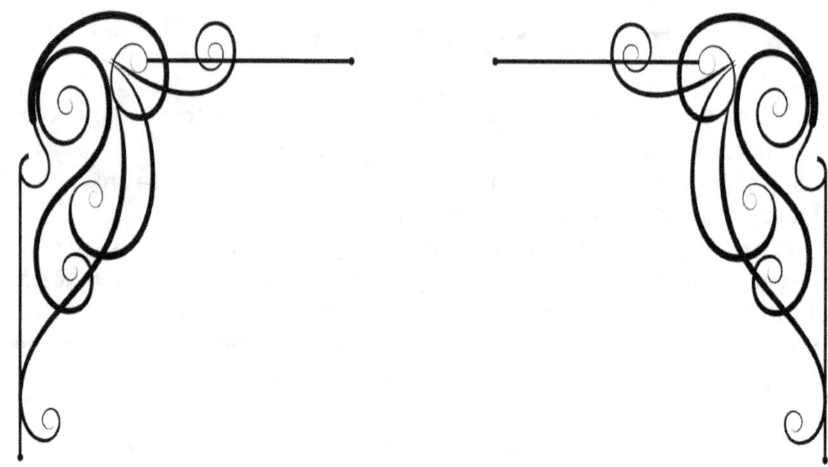

"Keep dreaming,
wishing,
and planning.

There's immeasurable
power in it."

~ Laura Smith

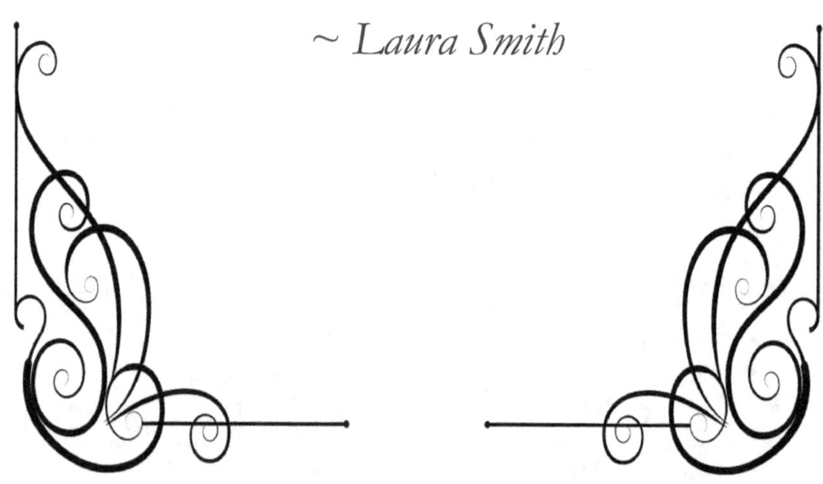

You want to view these as mini steps to your main goal. For example, if your main goal was to exercise more, spending ten minutes each day is a great way to start. Once you are in the habit of doing this increase the time by creating a new habit.

All of these smaller habits will take you about 21 days to achieve. Once you find you automatically eat that banana each day it is time to add the next one into the link. Before you know it, you will be well on your way to reaching your larger goal.

Saying your goals out loud to yourself is another great way to reinforce them in your mind. This will act as a reminder of what you want to achieve. Try this each morning while getting dressed or each evening after dinner.

Avoiding distractions

This is probably one of the biggest reasons why goals are never achieved. Life is full of distractions and yes, it can be so easy to get off track. You need to learn to stay focused.

Some of the top distractions which can be blamed for not reaching your goals is by always wanting to be perfect at everything you do. Being perfect is not necessary and you must be willing to accept that things will get in your way. But just because you get off track a bit it doesn't mean that you have to give up on your goal.

It's part of human nature to give into a craving, or to miss a workout class. What you do not want is to let this become a habit. When you are distracted just figure out a way of getting back on track quickly.

Stumbling through a difficult task at work is better than giving up because you can't execute it perfectly all the way through. You persevered and got the job done. Your boss will notice this and that can help especially if your goal is to move up within the company.

Being open minded is another way of how you can beat distractions. While you may have spent a lot of time on writing out and planning the path to your goal, be open and accepting of new ideas. If someone were to offer you help or guidance don't be closed minded and not listen to their advice. Remember that your way doesn't always have to be the one and only way! Be open to suggestions and be willing to try them out.

Along the same lines you should never be afraid or unwilling to reach out to others for assistance. If your progress is not progressing according to plan, then ask a friend or co-worker for advice. Many people are only too willing to help and are just waiting to be asked!

What all of this really boils down to is a mental fight in your head. You probably understand where I am coming from with this and you've probably experienced this feeling at some point or other.

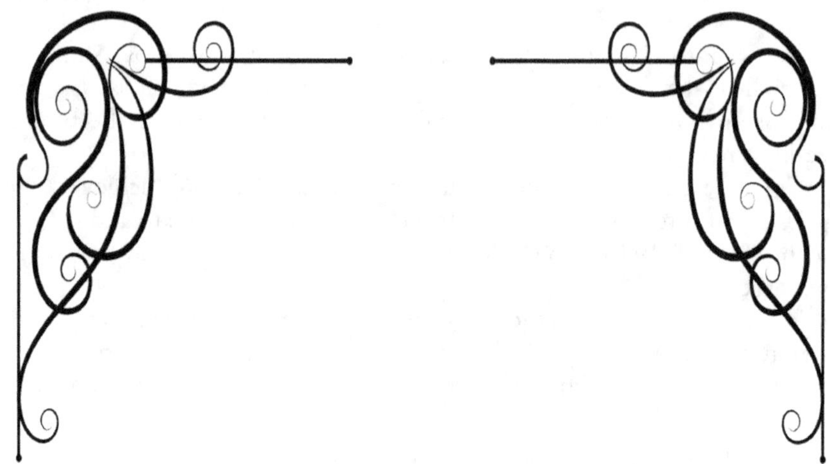

**"If it's important
you'll find a way.**

**If it's not,
you'll find excuses."**

~ Ryan Blair

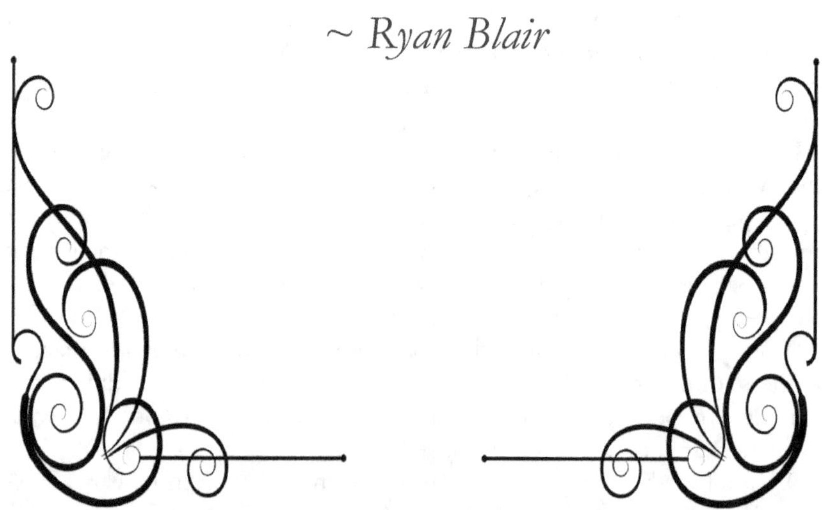

EXPECT AND PREPARE FOR SETBACKS

If you do experience a setback your first action is to not let your mind take over with a downward negative thinking. If you allow yourself to give up, you will never reach your goal. Plus, your belief in yourself will plummet and this is definitely not where you want to be.

Strive for progress, not perfection.

Whatever obstacle is standing in your way you want to make sure you find a way to deal with it. Your obstacle may just be negative comments from your family, co-workers or friends. Don't let other people's opinions become the obstacles that throw you off track. Burt Reynolds was once told to give up because he had no talent. Good thing he didn't listen! In fact, many famous people were told to give up on things and they refused to.

To handle a negative situation well you want to come equipped with positive thoughts. This is where using motivational quotes and affirmations can come in handy. They can help reinforce your belief in yourself.

If your obstacle is something different such as a time restraint, then look for ways to remove this new barrier. Maybe your exercise class has been rescheduled to a time that is inconvenient? See if there is another class you could take or consider joining a new gym if that is the only solution.

There are ways to overcome any obstacle or negative situation. Just be open-minded and look for ways to work around them. As much as we would all like to work towards our goals at a steady, uninterrupted pace, this is not always possible. Remember, where there is a will, there is a way.

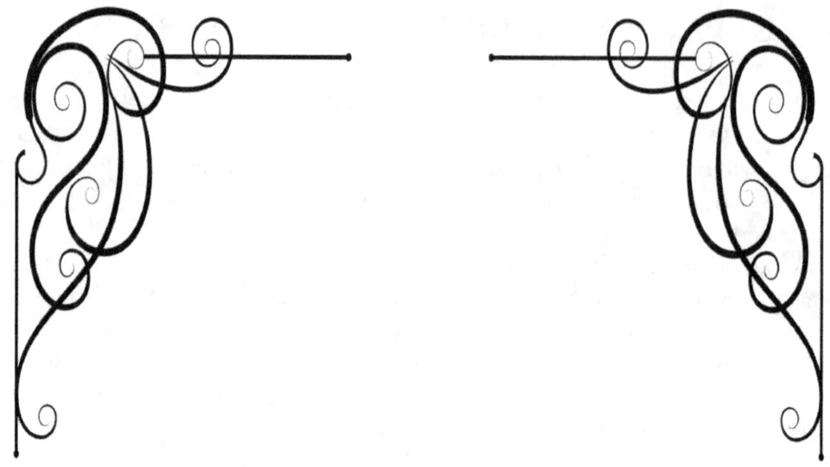

"Make a list of what is
really important to you.

Embody it."

~ *Jon Kabat-Zinn*

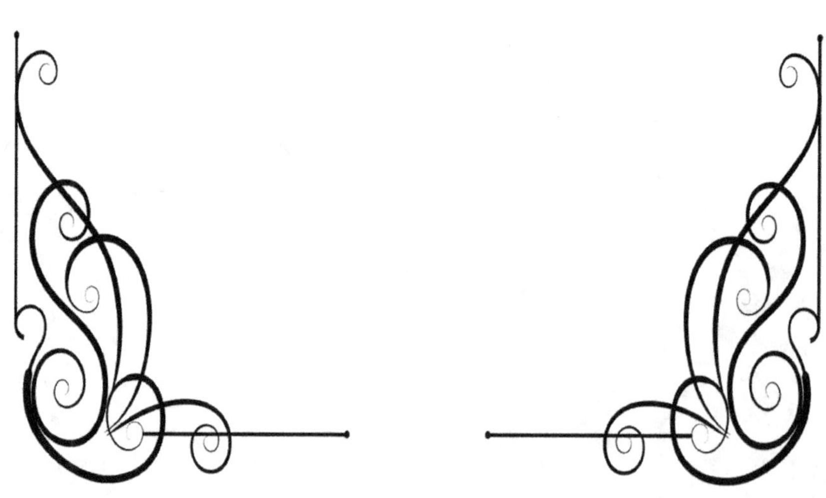

MAKE DAILY PROGRESS

It is important to make progress on a daily basis with your goals. While we talked about setbacks and interruptions here's some additional information that can help you stay in a positive mindset.

Your mind is an incredibly powerful tool and one that you want to enhance in any way possible. Even though you may feel that you are not spending enough time on your goal you want to look at the quality of how you spend the time you have.

What this means is that it's far better to spend 15 minutes totally concentrating on your goal, than to spend one hour where you are distracted by other things.

The time working on your goals is often referred to as mental engagement. Quite often it is much easier to spend time mentally working on your goal as opposed to putting in physical work. Included in this is time spent on visualizing where you want to be, or how you will look and feel once your goal is achieved. Of course, your thoughts have to be a concentrated effort to focus on your future results and not just a quick thought that passes almost immediately.

But where and how can you grab those few minutes to work mentally on your goal? If you are on a plane, for example, use this time for visualization or for planning out your next week's meals and exercise plan. If your goal is business related work on a marketing plan or go over a presentation or speech in your head.

If you wake up early one morning and can't get back to sleep, get up while the house is quiet and work on your goals. Once you begin to use your mental focus more, you will find it easier to set goals and reach them.

This will also help you concentrate and focus more on all kinds of tasks in both your personal and professional life.

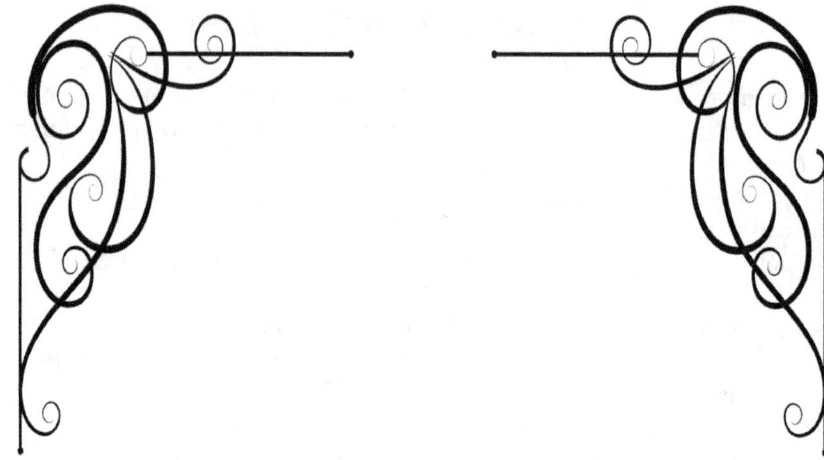

"Dream it.

Declare it.

Do it!"

~ Unknown

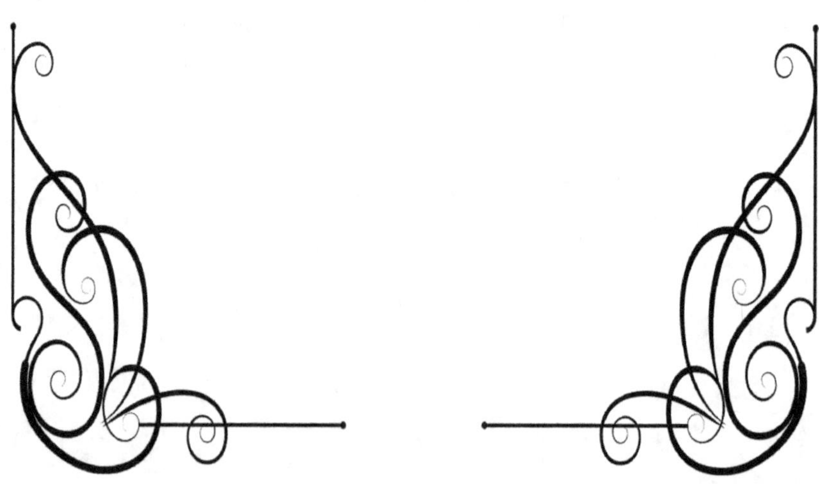

MAKE YOURSELF ACCOUNTABLE

For accountability to work you need to make your resolutions and goals known to other people. When you make a public declaration you immediately put yourself into the limelight. People are now going to expect to see results.

Think of places and people that you can declare your intentions to including:

- Post on Facebook or send out a Tweet.
- Write a note to friends and family.
- Make a pledge to your partner.
- Put up a sticky note on your fridge.
- Write on your blog.
- Email your list and announce your intentions.
- Create a short video and post it to YouTube.

What is accountability?

Accountability is an obligation or willingness to accept responsibility or to account for your actions.

To achieve your goals, focus on becoming accountable by declaring your intentions to at least one other person. You also want to be accountable to yourself. This involves having a positive mindset and setting your expectations to achieve your goals. If you expect to fail, you will. It really is as simple as that.

Understanding the personal accountability

Whether you are trying to stick to a resolution or reach a specific goal, it's extremely important to be true to yourself. Being personally accountable for your actions is something that everyone can learn. Use the following tips to achieve this, it is a key to the making your resolution personal revolution.

Being responsible involves your way of thinking and how you look at certain situations. A responsible person believes that their success or failure is up to them. Your first step, even before taking any action, is to commit to seeing your results. Believe you can achieve your goals. You must believe it before you can achieve it.

Most people are only too happy to take responsibility for all the good things that happen. When things go in the opposite direction it is much harder for people to admit responsibility. With your new goals it is important to acknowledge that you are willing to be 100% responsible regardless of the outcome, good or bad.

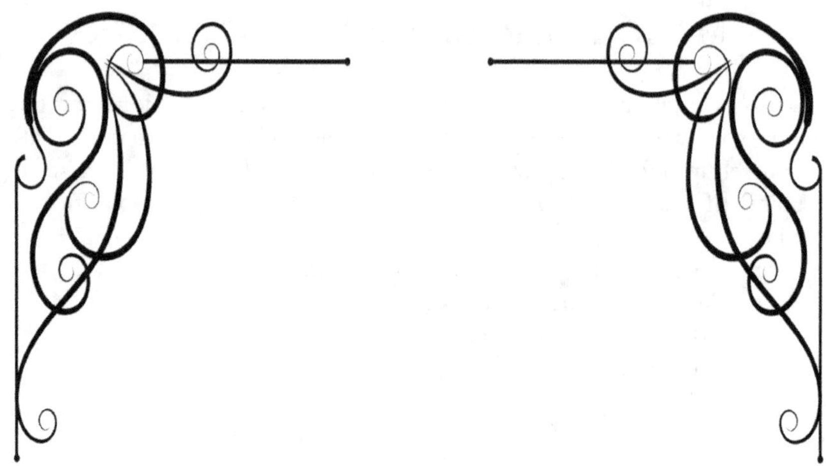

"At the end of the day we are
accountable to ourselves,
our success is a result
of what we do."

~ Catherine Pulsifer

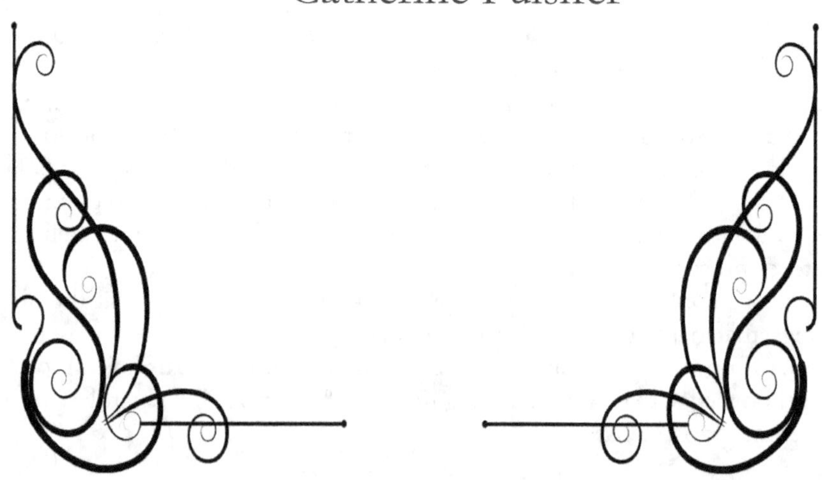

Stop living in the past. This is something that so many people do, and it's important to learn how to let go. What happened before is over and done. The past is past. You cannot change the outcome so learn to live with it. If you find yourself ruminating about the woulda, shoulda, coulda's in life, stop right now. From this moment on you need to think about how to deal with different situations as they present themselves, including obstacles, challenges and slip-ups.

Self-empowerment

You want to learn how to make things happen in your life. This can be accomplished by becoming self-empowered. It involves taking the actions and accepting the risks necessary to achieve your goals. Don't get into the habit of waiting for things or people to come to you. Instead, be proactive. Go out there and chase down your goals and dreams.

First, set your expectations. Being self-empowered means know what results you expect from your goal and you know what is expected of you to achieve those results. Before committing to any goal make sure you understand the risks and rewards. This applies to job related goals and expectations your employer may be setting for you. Some goals may not be worth the costs of success.

When setting new goals always keep in mind that your goal may require additional time and effort from you. This could cause a conflict in your scheduling or with other regular commitments. It is your choice to say no and you should do so. There is no point in overwhelming yourself with too many tasks, remember there are only so many hours in the day.

Be proud of your accomplishments and it never hurts to sing your own praises. Just don't overdo it.

Personal accountability and integrity

Your personal accountability is defined as the portion that comes at the end of your goal setting. Accepting personal accountability is being willing to accept the outcome of your choices and actions. So instead of blaming others for your results you accept that the blame falls on you, regardless of whether the outcome affects you personally or causes issues for other people.

Telling the truth is part of your personal integrity. Own your mistakes. When things go wrong don't lie about it or try to cover it up. You are the only one who can truly hold yourself accountability. There's no point in cheating or lying to yourself. You will only end up hurting yourself in the end. Don't lie to yourself. When you don't believe in things yourself no one else will either.

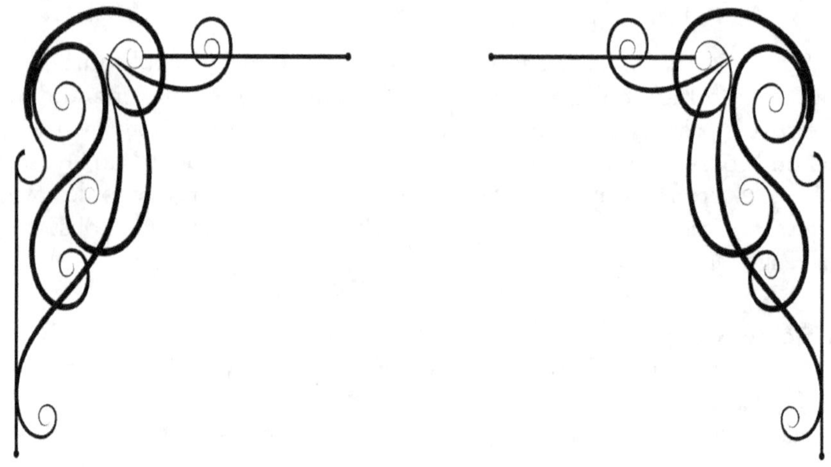

**Accountability is the glue
that ties the commitment to
the result.**

~ Bob Proctor

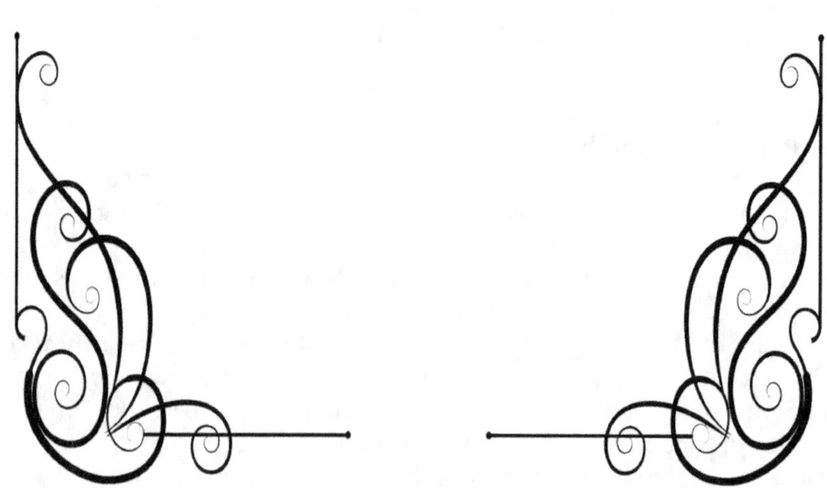

When you see that your goal is going off course look for the reasons why. Try to discover the problem. It could be something that you are doing and if so ask yourself how you can do it differently.

Unfortunately, too many people lack personal accountability in their personal and professional lives. Be willing to accept responsibility and take accountable for your actions. When you do, you will have become a much stronger person.

Accountability in the workplace

Accountability in the workplace means taking responsibility to complete the tasks or assignments that you were given by your employer. This includes showing up to work on time and fulfilling your obligations. If you are constantly late or underperform your job you must be willing to accept the consequences.

Some examples of workplace accountability are:

- Arriving for work on time.
- Completing your tasks correctly and in a timely fashion.
- Taking responsibility for your duties.
- Performing at a consistent level.
- Working in teams to help the company reach its goals.

Every employee is required to take accountability for their actions at work. It doesn't matter if you are in an entry level position or senior management. Everyone is expected to work together and help the business be successful. That means everyone is working towards a common goal. The end result is a company that becomes more productive, efficient and profitable.

Employers can use certain tactics and devices to keep track of employee accountability. This can be as simple as having employees swipe a card when arriving at work or by using a more complicated system such as retinal scanners. This allows the employer to track employees who arrive for work on time and identify employees who are constantly late.

Many businesses will use the SMART goal setting method for their employees. This provides each employee with goals that they need to be accountable for. This method has been shown to increase productivity on a large scale.

Incentive programs are another great workplace accountability method. Groups of employees will work together to achieve a pre-defined goal. They are then rewarded upon successful completion.

Employers can help their employees become more accountable and successful by having good time management procedures in place. One big reason why employees often fail to be accountable is due to poor time management. Helping employees get organized and stay on track is a win-win solution for everyone involved.

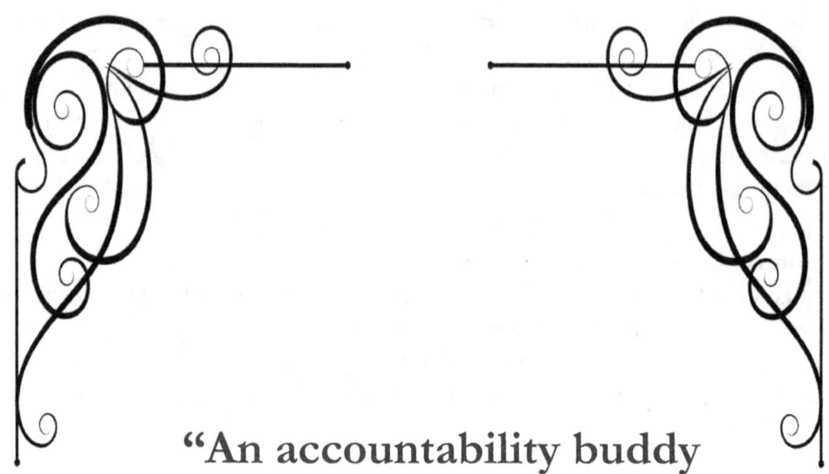

"An accountability buddy

can smooth out the bumps

along the way and travelling

together makes the journey

more enjoyable."

~ Carol Stockall

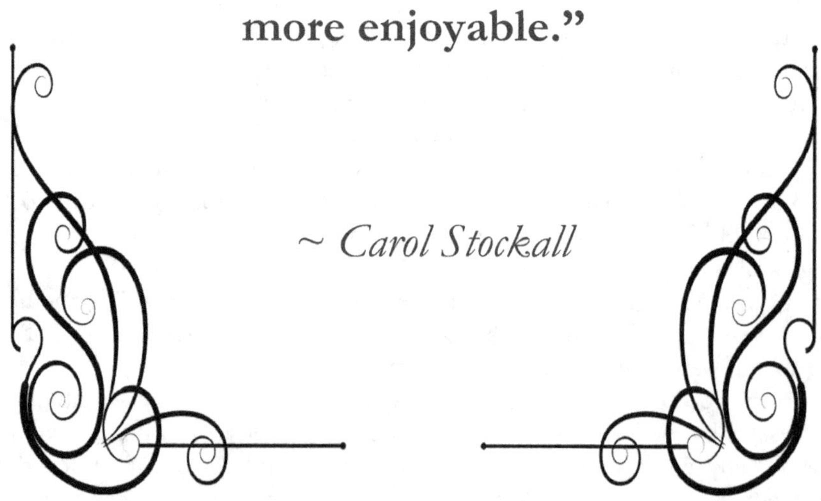

When an employee's progress is monitored, their productivity levels increase along with their accountability. It is part of human nature that when you know someone is watching you, you put in that extra effort. While monitoring helps, employers must also share their results in the form of progress reports for individuals as well as for the company as a whole. It's important to celebrate and leverage your strengths while working to improve your weaknesses.

Remember that personal accountability in the workplace encompasses many different aspects. It means doing the very best job you can, helping out when necessary and becoming a leader in certain areas.

If your goal is to secure a promotion, then taking on more personal accountability is going to have a positive effect on your chances. By demonstrating what you are capable of your manager or supervisor will have no option but to notice your actions.

Being accountable

You can be accountable by telling people about your goals. This includes telling your family and close friends what your new goals and resolutions are for the coming year.

Other ways to inform people of your goals include mentioning it on your website or blog if you have one. If you have a mailing list, you can let them know about your new goals.

Another great way to become accountable is to mention it on your social media sites. By doing this you are publicly declaring your intentions to improve an area of your life, or to get a goal achieved. You may also find that once you have stated your goals, others will be willing to join you on your journey.

Get an accountability partner

When you are accountable to one specific person you will find that your motivation stays high. You may even feel uncomfortable at first going this route and opening up to someone.

Eventually you will find that you enjoy your meetings and setting goals and deadlines. There will be times you don't get things done, and that is fine, you will still need to account for any delays. This can often help open up gaps or holes in your plans.

What is an accountability partner?

The term accountability partner has been around for a long time and it was often used by Christians who wanted to keep each other accountable for their behaviors. Nowadays this term is associated with finding someone that can help you stay on track to meet your goals.

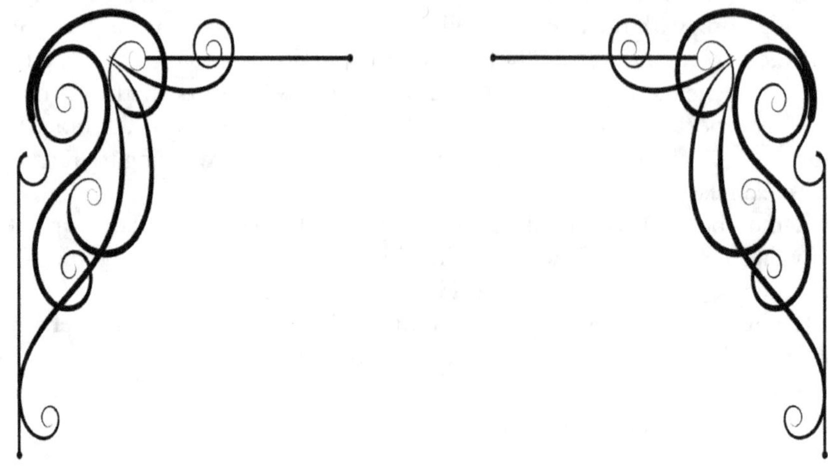

"Only put off until tomorrow
what you are willing to die
having left undone."

Pablo Picasso

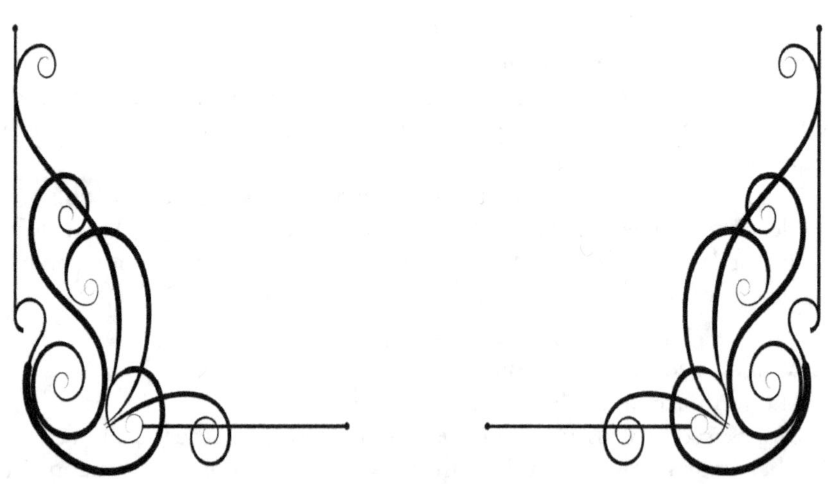

When deciding if an accountability partner would work for you remember that this is not the same as hiring a coach or mentor. Accountability partners are normally on an equal level and you both agree to help each other out.

No matter how large or small your goal is each person is going to hold the other accountable. Having an accountability partner is not a sign of weakness; in fact, it is the total opposite. You have the strength to know that you need to take action to improve your productivity. Many successful businesspeople have accountability partners who they talk to each week.

The main benefit of having an accountability partner is that you have to learn how to set specific goals each time you meet. Your goal may be to write five email messages for your autoresponder, or you may want to limit the amount of coffee you drink over the next few days.

An accountability partner can help you open your eyes to objections that you may have been too stubborn to see. Sometimes you can be trying so hard to achieve something that you lose total focus or even become out of touch with reality.

Your partner is going to help you stay motivated and this is a huge deal. Lack of motivation is one of the top reasons why goals and resolutions are not met. This applies to both your personal and your business goals. An added advantage is that your partner may be more understanding of your business situation than a close friend or even your partner.

How to find your accountability partner

Choosing a suitable accountability partner is not something that you want to rush into. You need to choose a partner that you feel comfortable with. You do not want to feel embarrassed about sharing your fears with your partner, it is important that you are honest with each other.

When looking for a partner you want to understand the purpose you have in mind for them. Make sure that you share this with them as well. It always helps to make notes on the qualities that you are looking for.

You may discover that your accountability is someone that you already know, or you may want to connect with a totally new person. Look around you and see who your business and personal acquaintances are. Are there any possible candidates there?

If not, you may have to look outside of your social circles. If you are looking for a business accountability partner turn to forums and groups that you belong to. Many forums have specific sections for people looking to connect with an accountability partner. You can always post a thread asking the group if anyone has interest in partnering.

You may have certain qualities that you are looking for, make a note of these if you do, so that you can easily compare your responses. Some qualities people look for include, gender, age, skill set, geography, and the overall logistics of getting together on a regular basis.

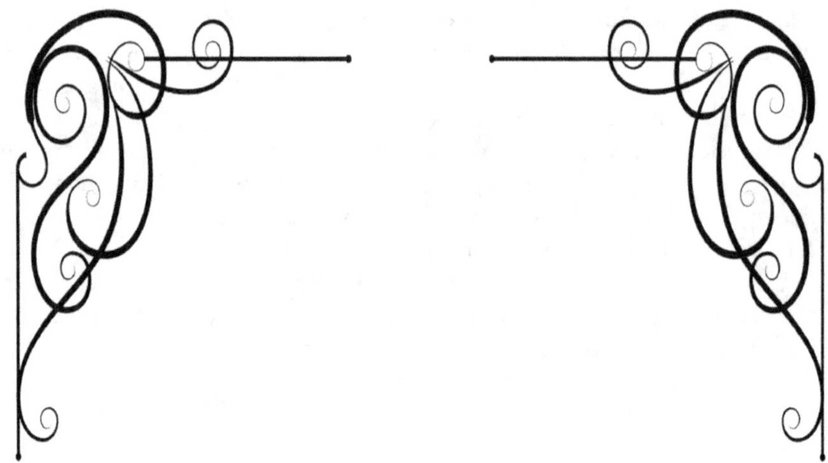

"Nobody can go back
and start a new beginning,
but anyone can start today
and make a new ending."

~ Maria Robinson

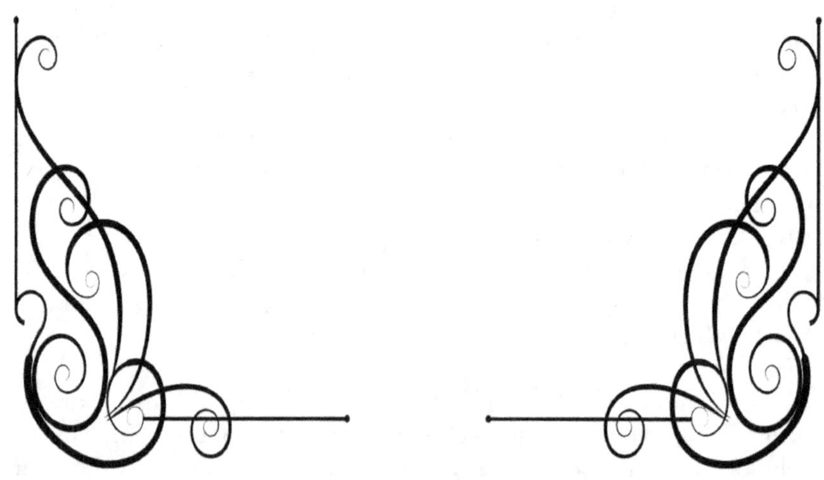

Accountability meetings

Once you have selected your partner you can start to set up your accountability meetings. Your first step is to arrange a convenient time for you both, this includes the day and time and the frequency that you want to meet.

Many partners like to start out with weekly accountability meetings and then move to bi-weekly or even monthly. As your meetings progress you will soon discover what suits you both best. You may prefer one longer meeting less often or you may wish to hold shorter weekly meetings.

Some business professionals only feel a need to connect with someone once or twice a year while keep motivation levels high by having a quick check-in with their partner each day.

Your agenda for each meeting depends on your goals. You want to spend the time discussing any obstacles or struggles that you may be having. During the week you should make a note of anything that you want to discuss with your partner. This way you won't waste any time during your meeting.

At the end of the day your accountability partner will help you with:

- understanding your task
- accepting your task
- setting a deadline for it to be done

You must also be prepared to accept responsibility for not meeting your deadline and explaining this to your partner. If you fail to reach your goal for whatever reason it is important to share the reason with your partner. They may be able to help you uncover a better course of action for reaching your goal. Of course, sometimes life just happens, and priorities must be set. But don't get into the habit of finding excuses for not achieving your tasks and goals.

You must always be willing to take ownership for your actions.

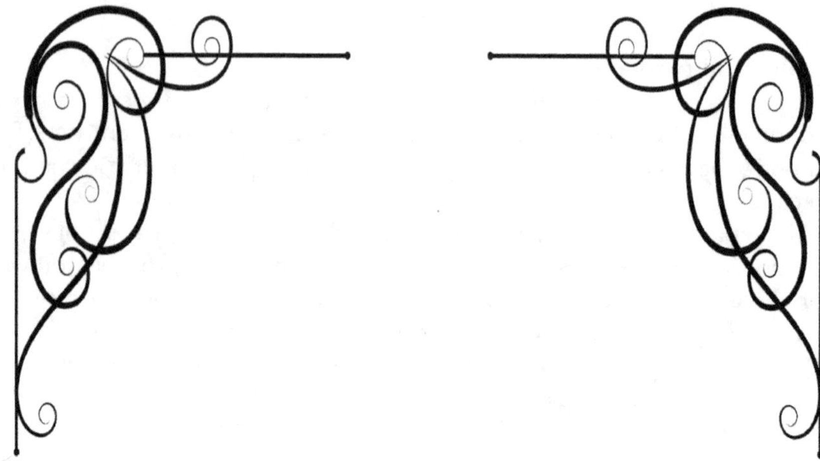

"Accountability breeds response-ability."

~ *Stephen R. Covey*

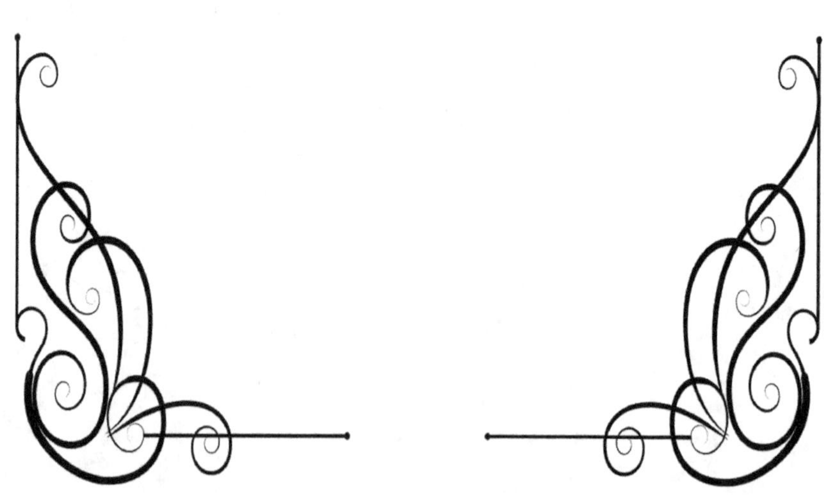

BENEFITS OF AN ACCOUNTABILITY PLAN

When you have an accountability plan in place there will be certain benefits that you will see including:

- Less worry, because knowing that you have a partner and you are finally taking action and making daily progress towards your end goal you can relax. You will accept that you are doing your best each and every day.
- With the perspective of your accountability partner you will discover other opinions and you may be more objective and open to considering different options.
- Your mind will focus more on your goal with the contribution of an accountability partner and priorities may become more apparent.
- Shared strategies for success will help you find more effective ways to deal with friends, family, and others while you move towards your goal.

Of course, with any benefits there is usually a downside as well. Your major problem with an accountability plan is simple, it is hard to do! You are opening yourself up to take advice and direction from another person. You must be prepared to not always like what you hear.

While it is important to share with your partner be careful not to compare yourself with your partner. Other people may progress at a different pace and in different directions. Make sure you compare yourself to yourself. Work your action plan not someone else's.

Once you learn how to be personally accountable your stress decrease and your productivity will increase. People who are not accountable to themselves are normally dissatisfied, unhappy at work and at home and they are just not happy with who they are.

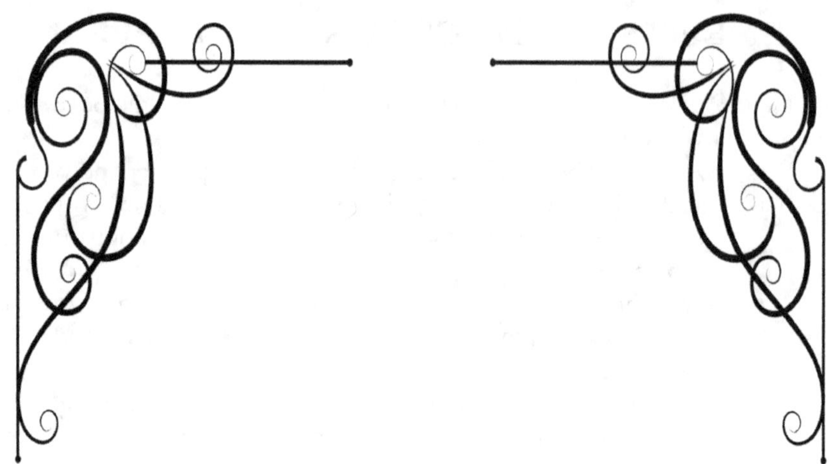

**"Accountability separates
the wishers in life from the
action-takers that care enough
about their future to account
for their daily actions."**

~ John Di Lemme

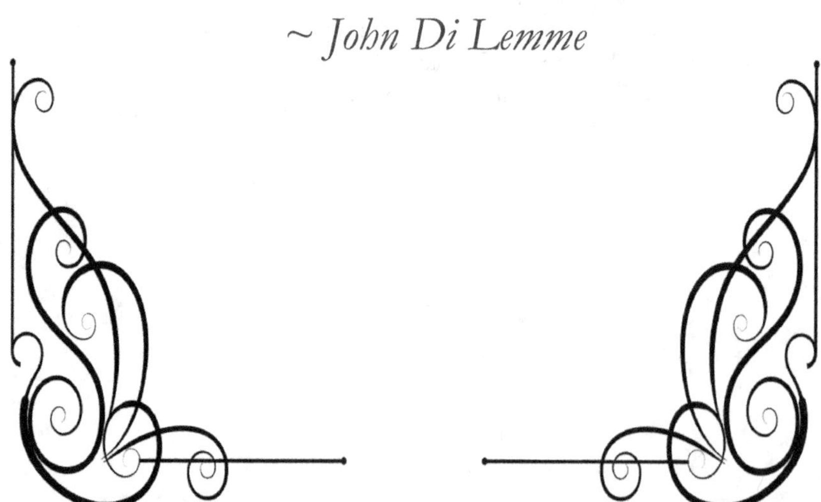

PART THREE:
STICKING TO YOUR GOALS

MAKE AN ACTION PLAN

Create a plan of action and stick to it.

You can do this my writing out a list of action steps which need to be done on a weekly or daily basis. Action steps are often referred to as actionable steps because they are something you have to do. This means writing out a plan with steps that require specific, measurable, do-able action. As this is a basic requirement for practically any goal let's look at this area in more depth.

Action steps can be added to a daily to-do list or inserted into a daily planner. As each action step is completed cross it off your list. If something is left as incomplete, make sure you add it as a priority the next day and get it done before starting on anything else.

By including both personal and business items you will find that you can balance out your schedule. With planning it is possible to create a solid balance in your life.

You can apply these same ideas to other types of goals including weight loss, exercise or working on improving your mind set. Create a detailed list of steps which you can accomplish each day. Examples for weight loss are:

- drink 8 cups of water
- walk for 20 minutes
- eat 2 servings of fruits
- include 2 veggie choices at lunch/dinner
- sleep 7 hours
- avoid sugar
- make healthy choices

This can help you stay motivated and keeps your whole approach to losing weight more manageable. Even if you only check off five out of the seven choices you are making progress and that is what is so important to remember. You can keep track of your progress in various ways including by creating lists, using a planner or using sticky notes

Create deadlines by setting dates and times to your goals. When you set a date and time to your goal you immediately make yourself more accountable. Instead of having a vague goal with no end in sight you now have a timeline. It can even help to write your deadline on a sticky note and place it in your bathroom, your kitchen fridge or stick in on your computer monitor. This way you have a daily reminder staring you right in the face.

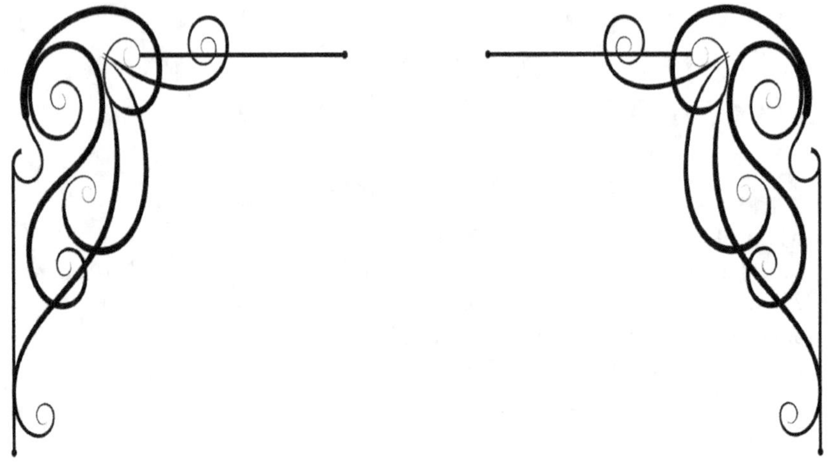

"Every choice you make has
an end result."

~ *Zig Ziglar*

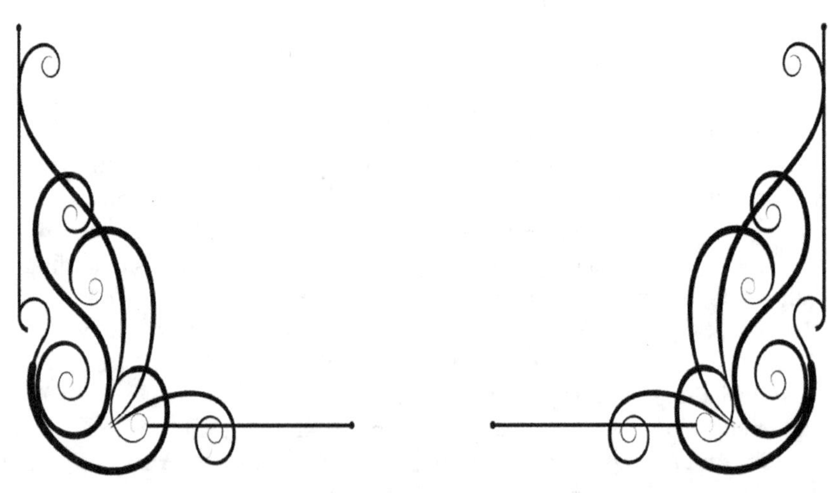

Announce your goals publicly. This helps to reinforce your goals in your own mind and makes you accountable to yourself, your friends and family and to everyone you have announced it to. Accountability creates expectations. When you know people are expecting something from you, it can help to spur you into massive action.

Using an accountability partner is the perfect way to stay on track and stay motivated. Don't forget that you can partner up with different people for different goals. Quite often losing weight or starting a new walking regimen is easier with a partner. If you know your friend is waiting for you at the end of the street every morning at 7:00am you are less likely to miss your walk.

Plan for the unexpected. If you plan for the unexpected common obstacles won't become roadblocks. Instead of using these things as an excuse you'll have a strategic plan for to overcome challenges.

To do this successfully you may want to fill in the blanks in the following phrase, if ___________, then _________.

Some examples are:

If my meeting runs late and I can't get to the gym, then I'll get up early tomorrow.

If I eat that piece of cake at the party today, then tomorrow I will go for an extra walk.

If my kids are sick and I miss my Yoga class, then I will just do my class at home the best I can.

Use small tools which can help you achieve your goals

Using tools to help you achieve your goals can be very effective. Today there are thousands of tools that you can use. Many of these are in the forms of Apps (Applications) that you can simply download to your computer, mobile device or phone.

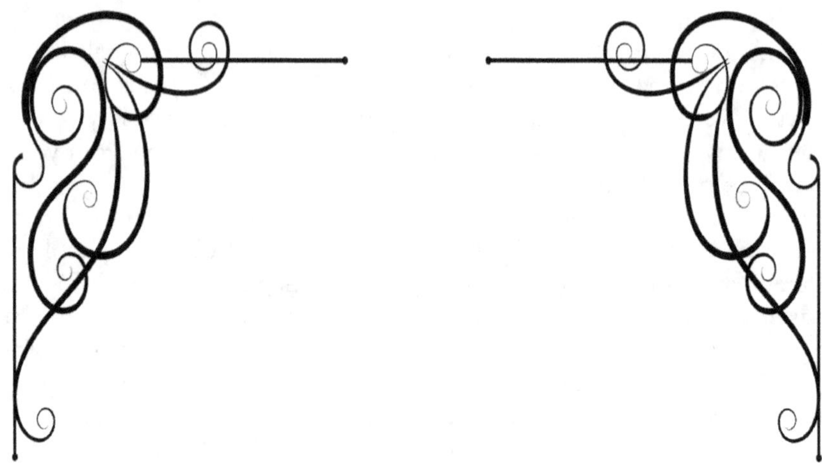

"When you come to the end
of your rope, tie a knot and
hang on."

~ Franklin D. Roosevelt

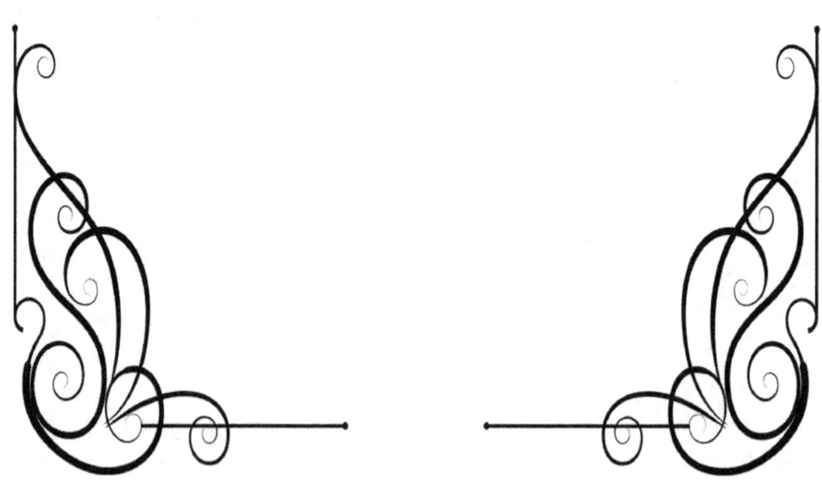

STICKING WITH IT

Sticking with a New Year's resolution for a whole year will not be without its struggles. A yearlong journey is inevitably fraught with numerous obstacles and many ups and downs. There may even roadblocks that require detours. Sticking with it is where the rubber meets the road. This journey will require both grace and grit.

Grit

Angela Duckworth's New York Times best-seller *Grit: The Power of Passion and Perseverance* refutes the idea that success is solely based on innate talent or genius. She says comes from grit, which she describes as an enduring combination of tenacity and passion. Duckworth draws on her own experiences and real-life stories of ordinary people and high achievers in business, teaching, and sports who pushed through their struggles to achieve their goals. She believes that grit can be learned. Grit is the muscle of inner strength. It's the strength you develop when you exercise the willpower to stay on track and keep moving towards your goal.

Grace

Sometimes the best way to develop a bit of grit is to start with a bit of grace. Start by writing a list of all the things you are grateful for, all your previous goals that are now accomplished successes. Celebrate your success. Use the enthusiasm and positive energy to empower your future success. List the factors that were important in achieving past success. Then rinse and repeat those factors to duplicate your success in your new goal.

Affirmations

Affirmations are a way to train your brain to accept positive input and energy. Collect affirmations that appeal to you. If you can't find any you like, make up your own. Write them on a notepad and post the notes all over your home. Decorate your space with affirmation graffiti. If you can, post them in your work area. Make sure they are somewhere where you can see them frequently throughout the day. Make a habit to pause and read them. Make up your own affirmations. Some example you might use are:

- I believe in myself.
- I can do this.
- Day by day I am getting closer and closer to my goal.
- I know what to do and I am doing it.
- I have an action plan and I am taking action to reach my goal.

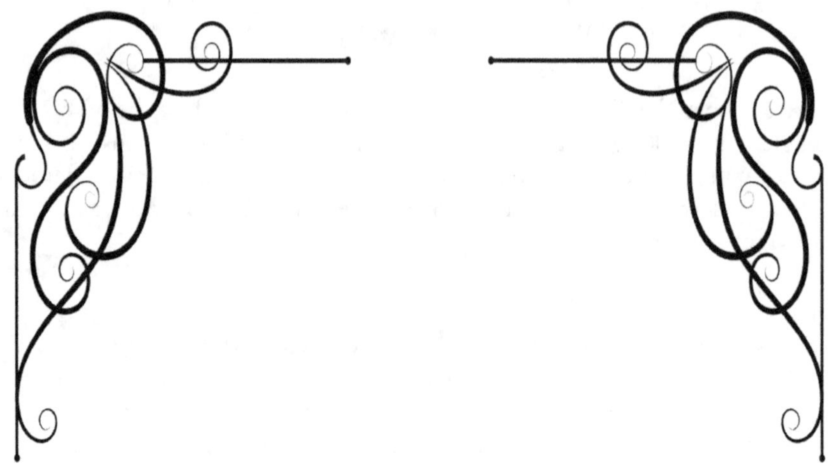

**"Dreams do come true,
if only we wish hard enough.
You can have anything in life if
you will sacrifice
everything else for it."**

~ J.M. Barrie

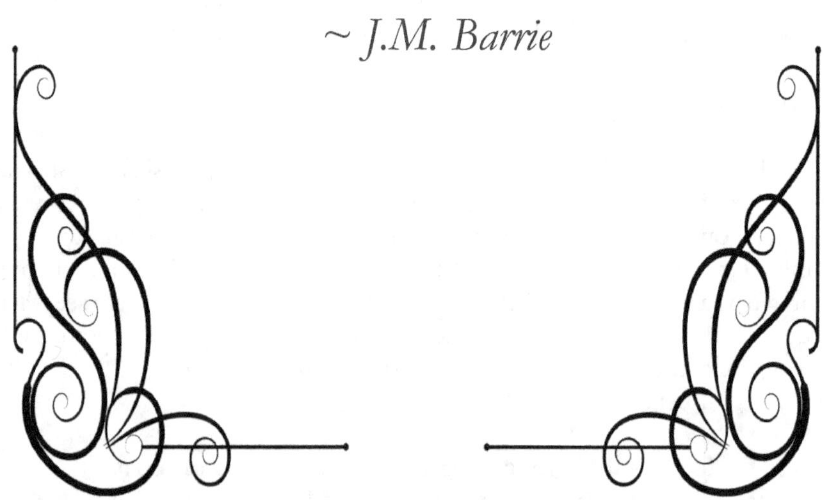

Visualization

Some goals may feel really challenging and you may find yourself wondering if you can achieve them. When this happens, it can be helpful to use visualization techniques to overcome your fear. Start visualizing how you will feel when you reach your goal. Make this visualization a daily habit. If your goal is connected to weight loss visualize how you will look in those new jeans or that new bathing suit.

Consequences of giving into temptation

It's so easy to miss a workout or eat that piece of cake or skip getting up early to work on your goal. This is when your willpower comes into play and it is when you need to dig down and find the strength to take action.

On those days when you feel yourself slipping, think about what the long-term result will be if you give in to your temptation. You can use the visualization method described above to visualize the consequences of giving in to temptation and then remember why you started this journey. If you let yourself eat that cake are you going to get into those skinny jeans by Christmas? Then ask yourself is it worth it or not. This strategy is often called playing the tape to the end. When you do this, you may find that you're not ready to let temptation get the better of you.

Even more important, when you do make a slip forgive yourself and get back on track. The faster you forgive yourself, the faster you get back on track. Learn from it and let it go.

Forums and groups

Joining a specific forum or group related to your goal can be really helpful. If your goal is to read more books, then joining a book club can be a huge help. If you want to write a book, then join a writer's group.

Weight loss forums can offer you support and additional tools for achieving your goals. It's always nice to chat with people who are struggling with the same things you are.

In fact, forums are so popular these days that you can almost find one for any goal or habit you are looking to make or break. Support forums exist for people dealing with drug addictions, smoking, and dealing with depression to name just a few.

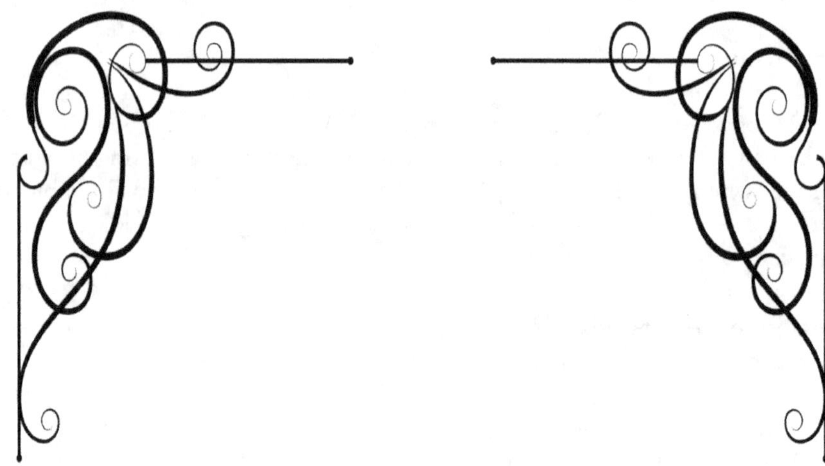

"Little by little
does the trick."

~ Aesop

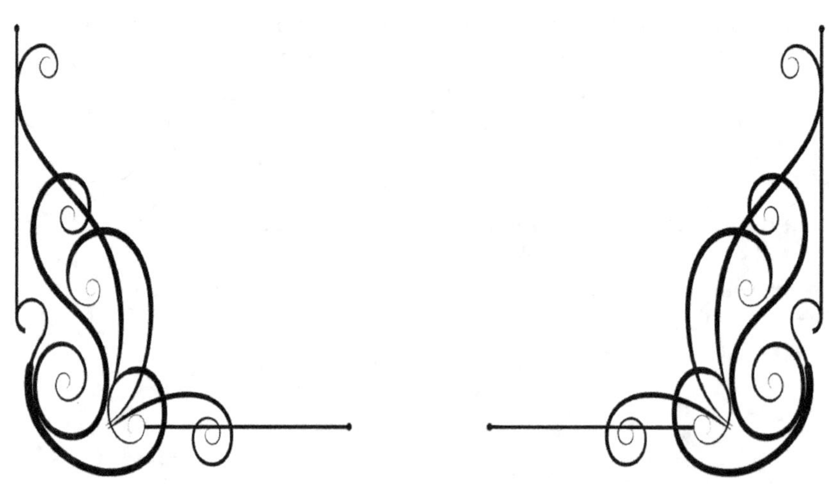

Take a challenge

Quite often challenges can be a fun way to accomplish your goal and a way to get other people involved with you. If your goal is to eat a healthier diet, then you could create a healthy eating challenge at work. If you blog, then blog about this topic and challenge your readers to do the same.

Challenges can vary in length. You can take a one-week, 21-day, or one-month challenge. In fact, a New Year's resolution could be considered a one-year challenge. Challenges can help with a variety of goals especially those centered around self-improvement; weight loss, exercise and learning a new skill or hobby. Get others to learn with you and the entire process becomes fun.

With the popularity of Apps, you can find ones that help you create goals. Some Apps will keep a running tally of your specific goals and evaluate your progress. For example, you can buy pedometers which keep track of your steps over a 30-day period. Once you determine what your daily average is then you can take this number and improve on it.

Bitesize your goal

Sometimes goals seem overwhelming, especially when they are big goals. Big goals can make you feel like you've bitten off more than you can chew. When a goal feels too big it is tempting to give up. But instead of giving up on your goal break it down into bitesize pieces. because they are so huge. Losing 50 pounds in a year can seem insurmountable as can training for a marathon or learning a totally new skill. But losing one pound a week seems doable. Similarly, marathon training is something that is built up over time.

It will be much easier for you to handle if you break down your goal into smaller, bitesize chunks. You can apply this method to any task that needs to be done in your life. If you have been putting off cleaning out the basement break it down. Select a day that you are going to do this task first and then assign a time period to it.

Say you choose the next Saturday for this, break the day into time chunks. From 8am – 9:30am you will start cleaning out the basement. Then allow yourself a break to go outside or sit and have a coffee. Repeat this process throughout the day and set a finishing time of say 4pm.

You can further break this down into the actual tasks you will be doing:

- finding empty boxes and putting them into the basement
- clean up tool bench
- check out kid's old toy box
- check on furnace, electrical box etc.
- create a family television area
- create a workout area

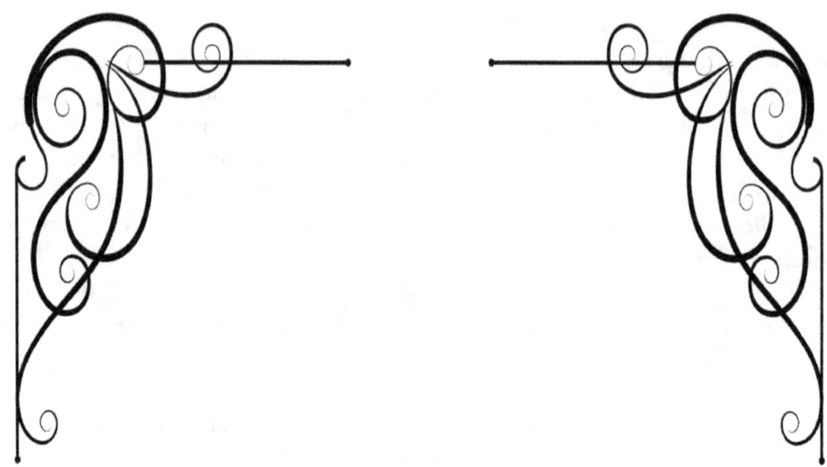

**"Accept responsibility
for your life.**

**Know that it is you who will
get you where you want to go,
no one else."**

~ Les Brown

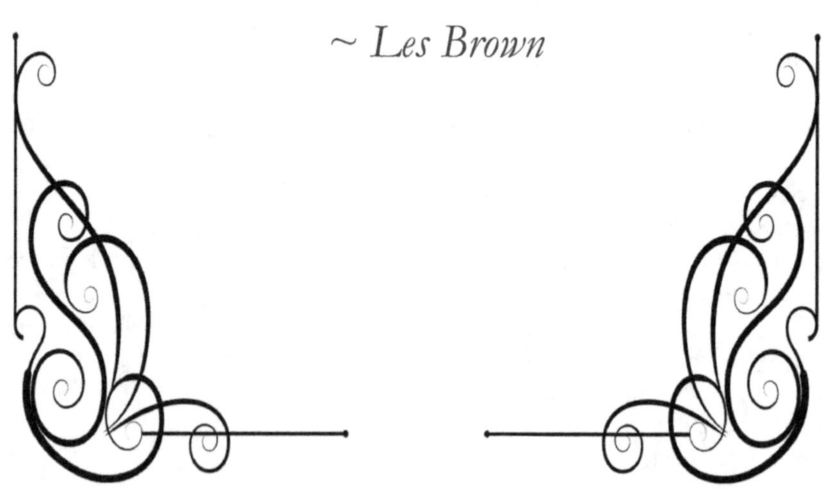

By doing this you are creating actionable steps that will help you get the task done. Take your list with you into the basement and cross off each job as it is completed. You'll feel great about just tackling the job and you will feel a huge sense of accomplishment once it is finished.

Book a day off

There is absolutely nothing wrong with having a day off from your goal. Your main concern here is that this day should be a day you plan in advance. You do not want to get into the mindset of allowing yourself a day off whenever you feel like it.

Choose a particular day in advance so that you can look forward to it and you can plan other activities. You may want to pick a day so that you can spend more time with your family, or you may prefer a day where you can just relax and recuperate.

Many weight loss experts agree that allowing a cheat day can be extremely helpful. You can have that piece of pizza or glass of wine without feeling guilty. Just remember you must set a start and end to your day off.

Stop thinking constantly about your goal

While we don't want you to lose your focus, often people tend to start over-thinking their goals. They allow their goal to become such a focus that they end up wearing horse blinders.

You need to start making conscious choices and then rely on yourself to continue making this choice. Things that fall into this realm include choosing whole wheat pasta and bread over white, taking the stairs instead of the elevator, parking at the back of the parking lot and more.

As you accomplish small segments of your goal, they become a habit, so you don't need to focus on them as much anymore. These things have become part of your regular lifestyle and not something extra that you 'have' to do each day.

Surround yourself with successful people

Stick with the winners. By surrounding yourself with successful people their success will automatically rub off on you. You have probably experienced this before in one way or another. If you are in a group of people who constantly complain you begin to do the same and you end up always feeling down and miserable. Think how you will feel if you surround yourself with people who want to get ahead in life? Successful people are great role models. Watch what they do and then see if that would work for you too. Successful people are great mentors. Listen to the advice they give and see if some of that would help you succeed too.

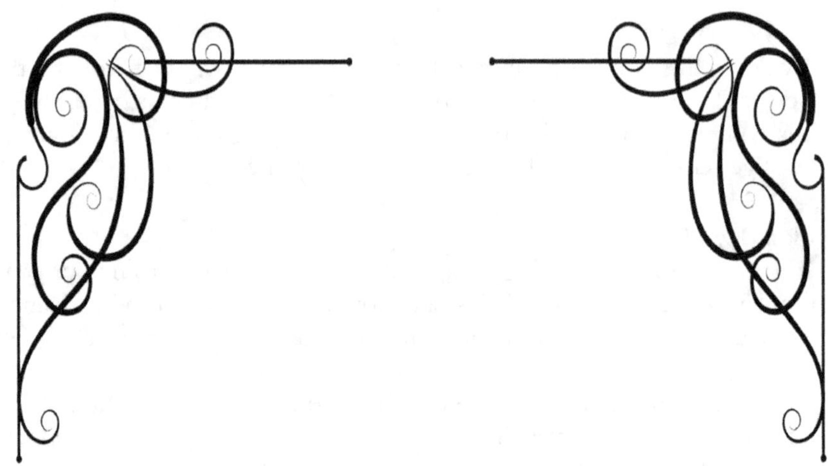

Every heart has
a hidden treasure.
A secret wish.
A silent dream.
A special goal to long for.

~ Jill Wolf

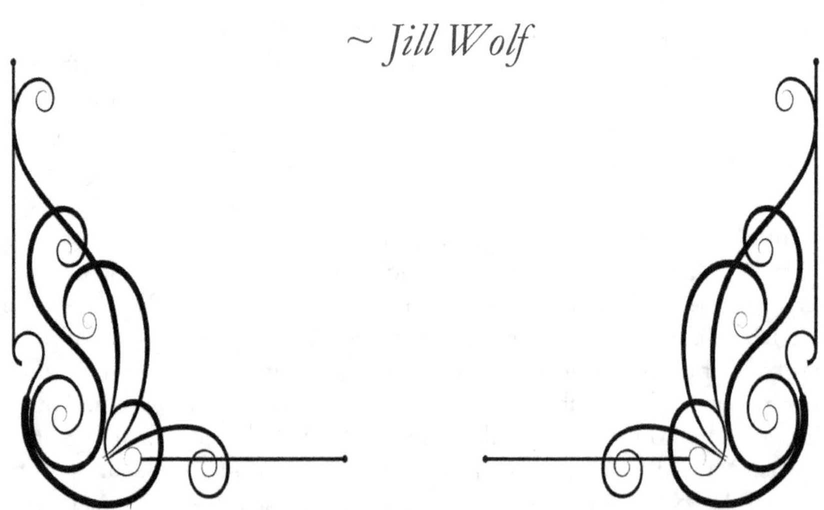

Reminders

Sometimes as you work towards your goal you may not feel as though you have come very far. This is exactly why it is a great idea to keep reminders. These can be in the form of notes, from writing in a journal or from a photo.

Keeping some type of reminder can be really helpful on those days when you are not feeling productive, and your end goal is nowhere in sight. Let's use weight loss as an example.

If you snap a photo of yourself when you begin your journey, every time you look at it you can see just how far you have come. Why not create a photo board of your journey so that you can track your progress?

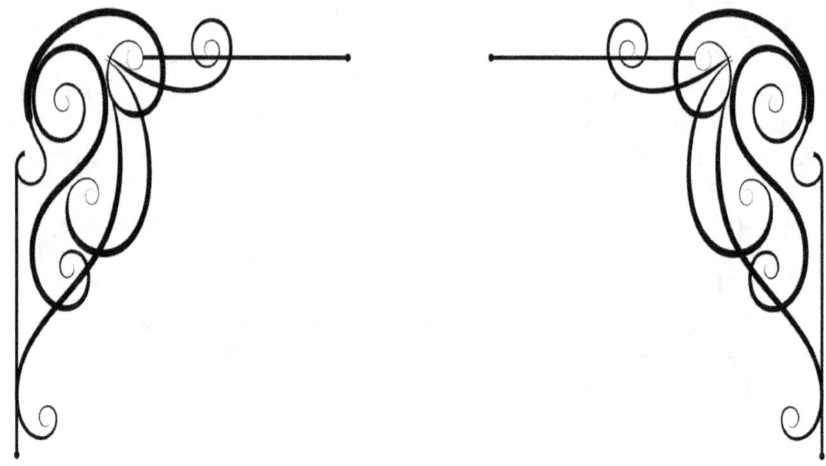

"**Stop doubting,
start doing.**"

~ Bianca Bass

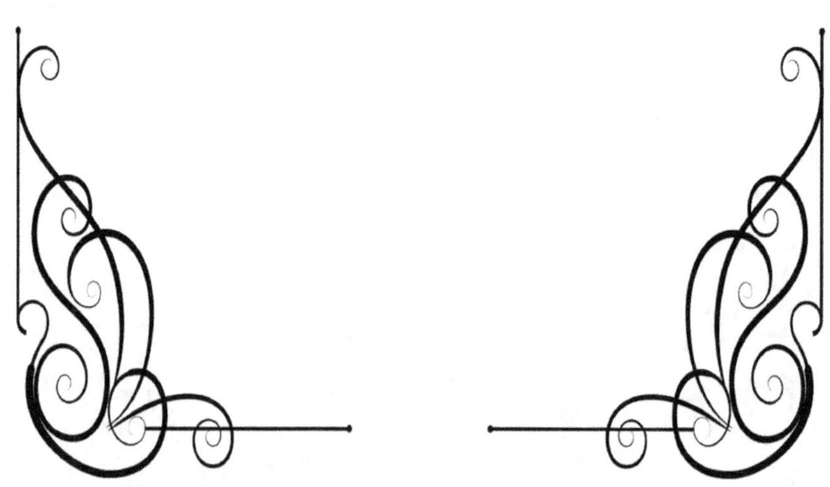

When your weight loss plateaus take another photo and then compare it with your first one. This should provide you with tons of motivation to stay on track and keep plugging towards your goal. The same applies if the scale isn't budging, try recording your measurements. You may find that instead of losing pounds you are losing lots of inches!

When looking back reflect on where you were and where you are right now! Congratulate yourself for making it that far and know that you can finish your journey.

You could also set a daily reminder on your phone that alerts you to an action step you need to take.

Planning

When you plan ahead you can eliminate some tough choices by having a prepared strategy to resist those sudden temptations when they arise. For example, if your goal is to create a healthier lifestyle set aside time each week to plan out your meals and exercise routine for the coming week.

This allows you to go out grocery shopping, for example, and select healthy choices. Each day you know what meals you are going to be having and even if you come home tired after a tough day at work; your meal choice is ready and waiting for you.

Planning in advice can become an activity that your entire family can enjoy together. Why not let the kids help plan on dinner per week? Or let them decide on a weekend activity that you can do together. Maybe they would love to go hiking or swimming with you.

Apply this tactic to any resolution or goal by writing down your plan for the week and even attaching a time to each item which you want to work on. This is a great way not to miss out on any school activities or to be available to help with homework. By doing this you can still enjoy plenty of time with your family and can map time to work on your own goals.

Nowadays there is a planner for almost everything. Browse the bookstores, office supply stores or online store and get a planner related to your goal. Find a planner that suits your goal and start planning.

Believe in yourself

There is no room for self-doubt when it comes to achieving your goals. Always remind yourself of what your goal is and get into the habit of telling yourself that you can and will do what it takes to achieve your goal.

By just believing that your goal is possible your success rate skyrockets. Even when that little voice pops into your head and says take a break, or eat that cookie, your belief in yourself lets you know you have the inner strength to resist and stay on track.

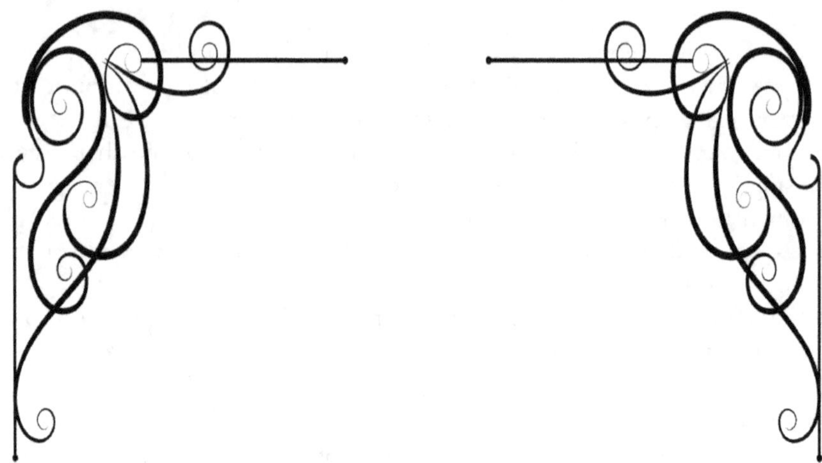

"It is good to have an end
to journey toward;
but it is the journey
that matters,
in the end."

~ Ernest Hemingway

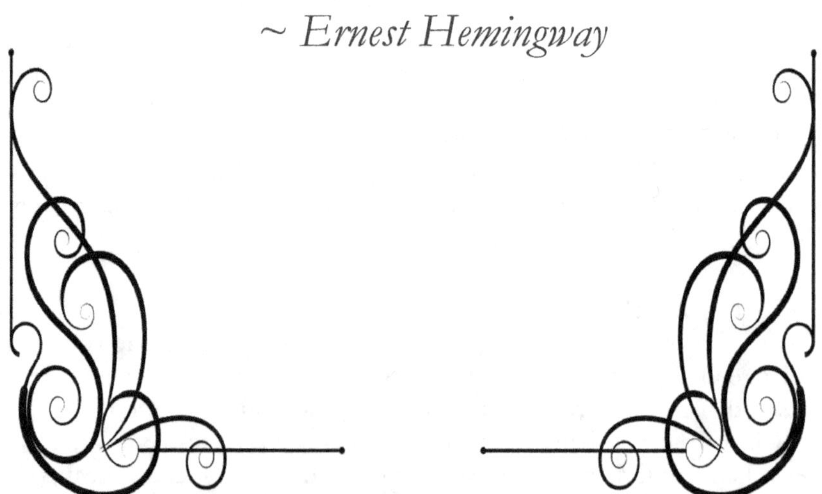

Remember you want to be like the little engine that was trying to get up the hill. Keep saying, "I know I can, I know I can," repeat it until you totally believe it.

Motivational Quotes

This is another great tactic which can really help you stay motivated and ready to take action each and every day. Find motivational quotes and affirmations that hold some type of meaning for you. Then simply place these quotes in places around your home and at work where you can read them several times a day.

You can use specific quotes pertaining to your goal or general goal orientated ones. This book is full of inspirational quotes you can use to get started. Search online for additional quotes and make a collection of favorites.

Ask for help

Never feel afraid to ask for help. No-one has to feel as they are superhuman and can take on all the world has to offer alone. The ability to ask for help is a strength not a weakness. Instead when you feel that you are struggling or are just feeling down and blue reach out and ask for help and advice.

Quite often when you do this you may be surprised by who jumps in to help you out. Most people don't always realize how many people are waiting in the wings to offer you help and guidance. They may even feel afraid about hurting your feelings, and this is why they have never offered their help before.

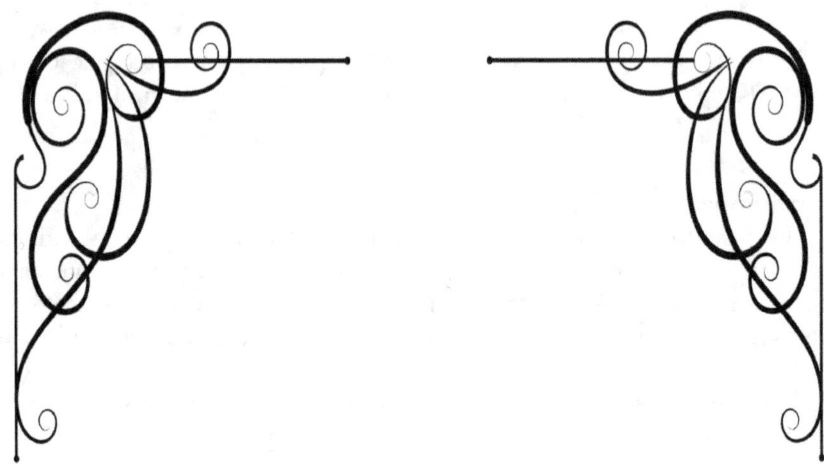

"Progress is impossible
without change and those who
cannot change their minds
cannot change anything."

~ *George Bernard Shaw*

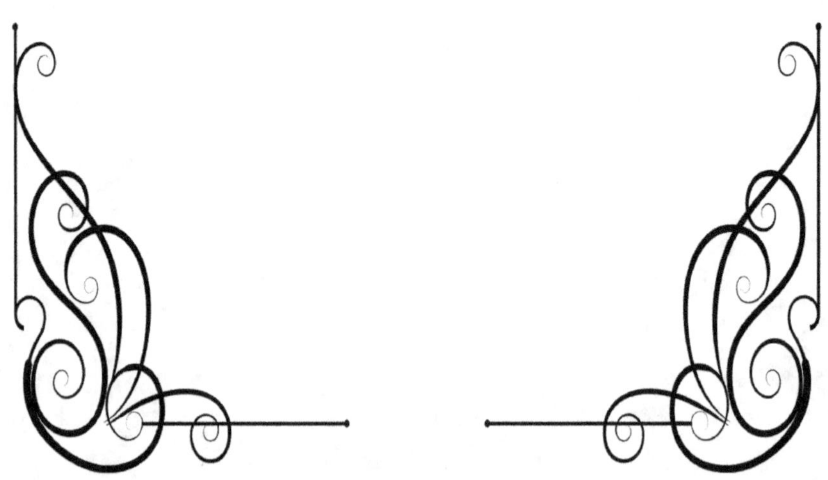

EXAMPLES OF ACTIONABLE STEPS

In this section will we look at some actionable steps that you can take to achieve your goal or resolutions. Below are some examples for actionable steps related to some of the most common New Year's resolutions.

Actionable steps for losing weight

1. start moving more every day
2. keep a food journal
3. parking your car further away at the mall or store
4. walking and not driving to the mailbox
5. use a pedometer to increase the daily number of steps you take
6. set a goal of 10,000 steps per day
7. include one fruit at breakfast
8. drink water each day
9. cut out soda one can at a time
10. reduce your salt intake
11. buy more fresh fruits and veggies
12. plan ahead for family gatherings and allow yourself to have a treat

Actionable steps for exercising more

1. schedule your workouts and make an appointment with yourself
2. set out your workout clothes before going to bed
3. use an exercise DVD or YouTube video for bad weather days
4. can't get to your workout class, do something at home
5. walk up and down your basement stairs more often
6. find a workout buddy
7. plan shorter exercise sessions if you are busy
8. take the stairs instead of the elevator
9. start doing push-ups against the wall or use your stairs
10. use an exercise ball to do sit ups
11. go swimming if your joints are sore or you have arthritis
12. rehydrate as you exercise
13. vary your workouts
14. moderate physical activity burns lots of calories - you don't have to go for the burn each session

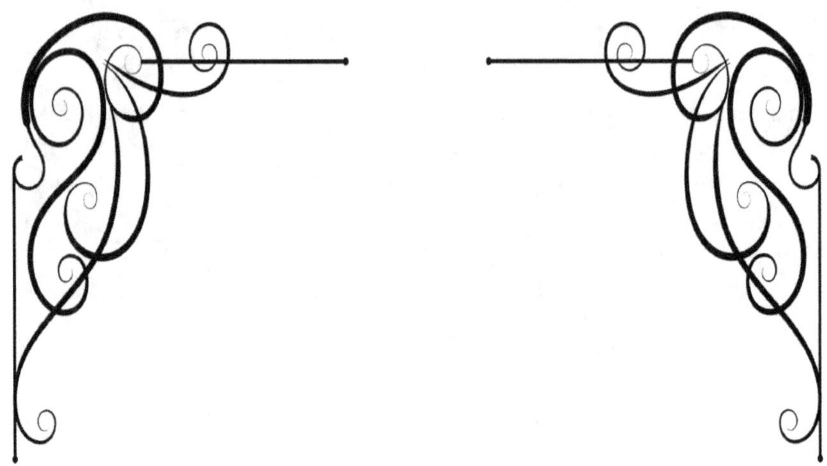

"If you're bored with life,
if you don't get up every
morning with a burning desire
to do things,
you don't have enough goals."

~ *Lou Holtz*

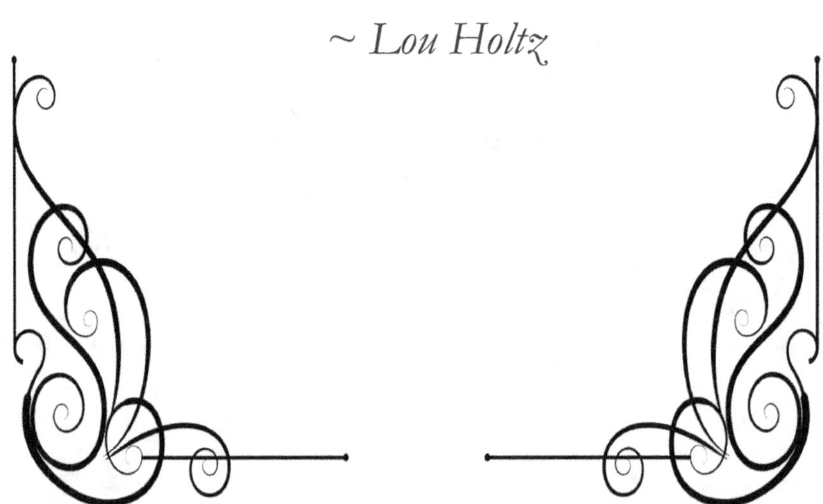

Actionable steps for quitting smoking
- remove temptations, get rid of your ashtrays, lighter and matches
- if your partner smokes, ask that they smoke outside
- don't visit your favorite smoking places
- avoid hanging out with friends that do nothing but smoke
- save the money you spent on cigarettes and treat yourself to something else
- start a new exercise program
- take up a new hobby
- stop thinking about not smoking as much
- post a list of your reasons why you want to quit smoking on the fridge, on the bathroom mirror, anywhere you'll see them often

Actionable steps for writers
- commit to writing a short blog post each day
- keep a daily journal
- learn to become a better writer
- set aside time to work on your writing each day
- find an accountability partner with similar goals
- do one small thing to move closer to publishing your book

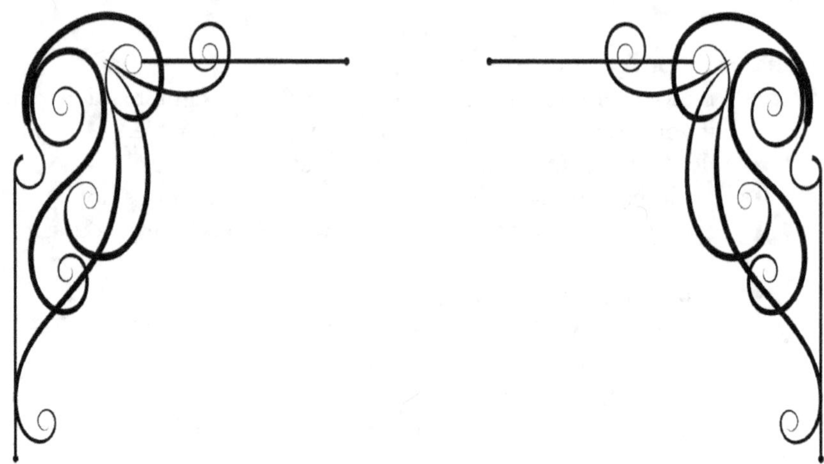

"**Character is the ability to carry out a good resolution long after the excitement of the moment has passed.**"

~ Cavett Robert

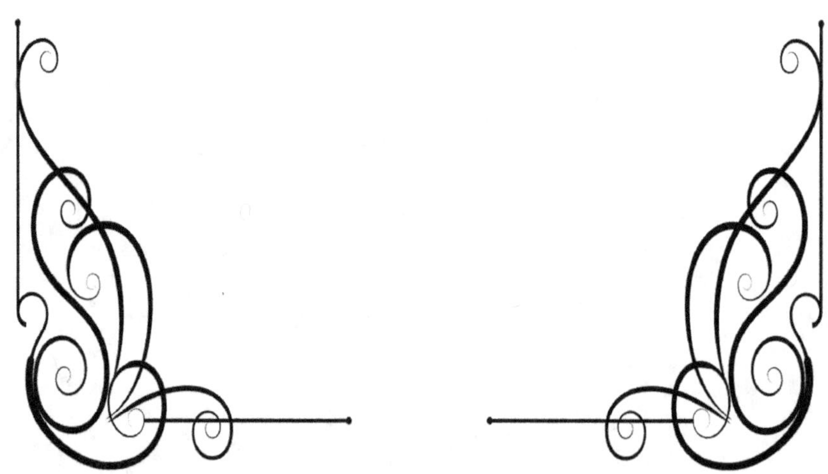

SETTING MILESTONES

Setting yourself milestones can help you stay on track with your goal. This is very true for those goals which you know are going to take you a long time to achieve.

A milestone is an action that helps you make progress towards your end goal. They can be defined as small steps or moves which can be used as measurements for success.

As you reach each milestone you want to take the time to evaluate your progress as well as seeing what difficulties or issues you encountered. This is an important learning process which can help you reorganize your approach, if necessary, to reach your next milestone.

Adjusting your milestone allows you to accept responsibility for your actions and to correct any mistakes or errors you may have made. It is important to understand and accept that unexpected things will crop up during your journey. Accept this and learn to deal with them and then move forward.

If you find your original goal is way out of whack, then create a new list of your challenges and redefine your goal as necessary. Being open to change is extremely important and it's also character building.

Look at each milestone as a mini goal which you need to achieve and set a date for you to reach it by. This allows you to celebrate those small successes. Ultimately, they will help increase your motivation and your staying power.

Set some form of measurable action so you can track your progress. Monitor your actions and take actions as necessary to stay on track. When you feel stuck then change things up. Add something new, find a new approach to tackle the situation. Don't just sit there and stay stagnant.

Try writing out your goals as though you have already achieved them. Use a future date and create your goal.

Example: It is December 24th and I fit into a size 8 pair of jeans and I love the way I have more energy and the way I look!

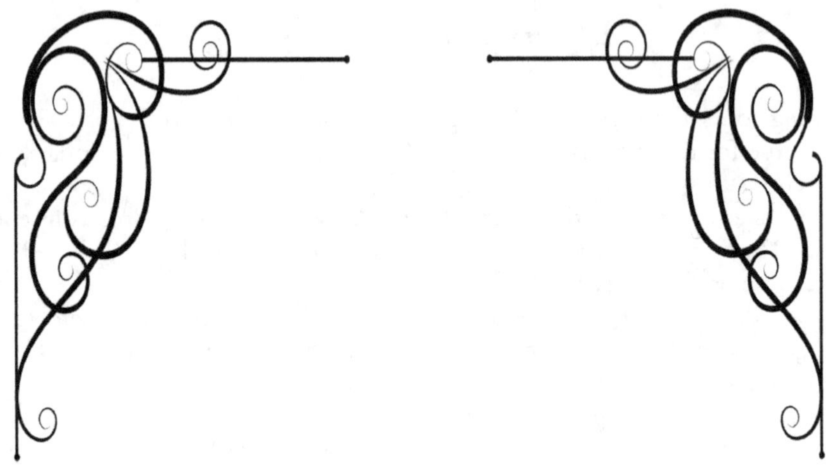

**"You are never too old
to set another goal
or to dream a new dream."**

~ C. S. Lewis

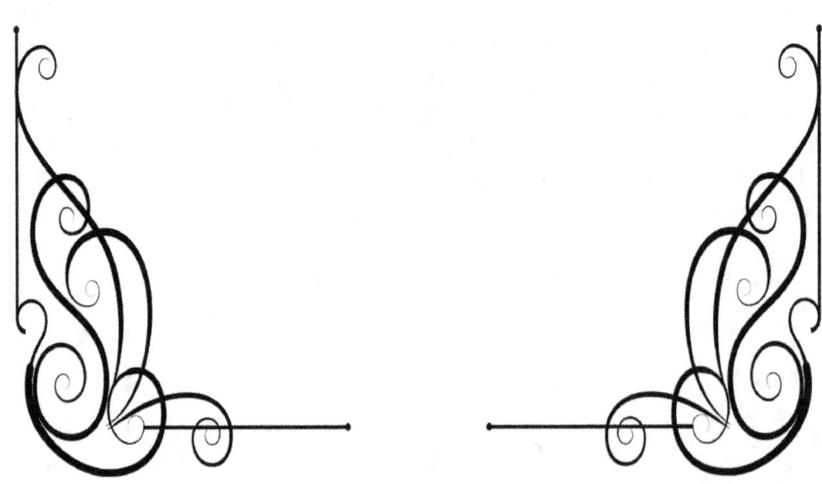

CREATE MONTHLY GOALS

If the goal you have set is one that will take you all year to complete you may want to seriously consider breaking it up into monthly segments. This will give you a new deadline for each month. Write out each goal for the end of every month and keep track of your progress. Create a simple spreadsheet for each month and the specified goal.

For example:

- By the end of the month I will be walking each day for at least 30 minutes.

Or

- By the end of the month I will be putting $25 each month into my retirement/business fund.

Each monthly segment should build from the previous month and lead you to successfully completing your main goal.

You could also sub divide this further by creating a weekly goal spreadsheet which further segments your actions. This is a personal choice, but some people find that they are more accountable and motivated when their plans are outlined in as much detail as possible.

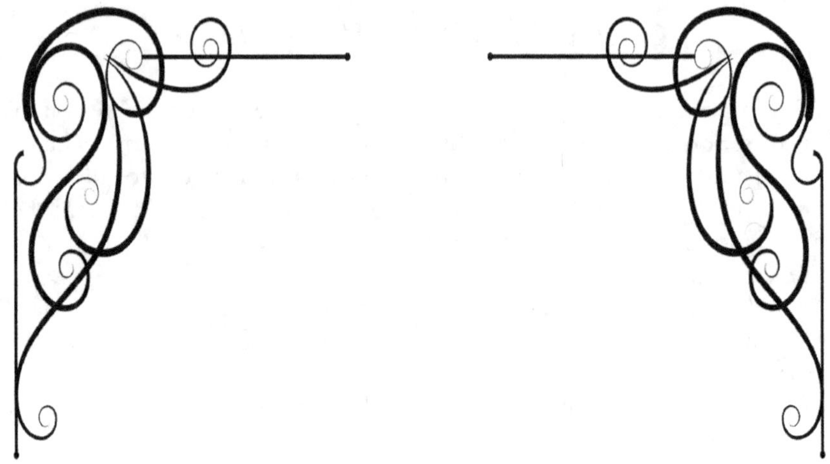

**"A year from now you will
wish you had started today."**

~ *Karen Lamb*

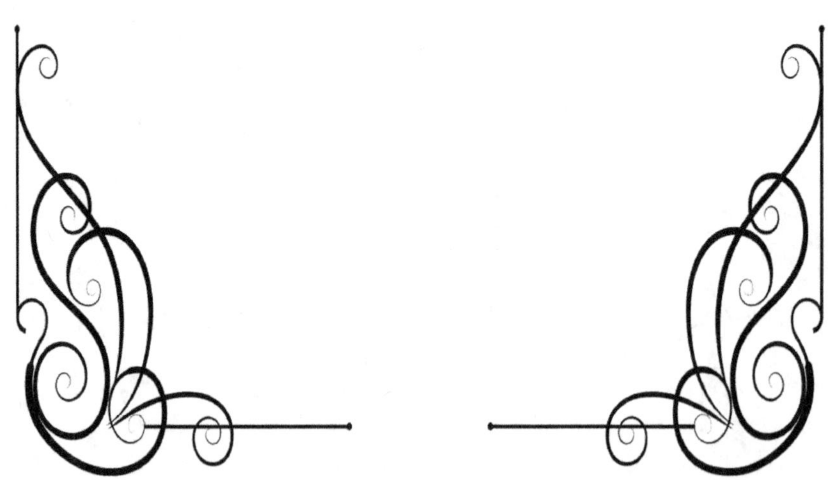

SAMPLES OF GOALS

In case you are still stuck at how to define your goal here are lists of some goals you can use. At the very least they should spark ideas which you can easily adapt for your own use.

Professional goals relating to career
- setting a date to become a manager
- reading 1 book by April on the best way to change careers
- submit your resume to 10 employers by February 1st
- self-publish that book that has been sitting on your hard drive
- outsource a task to a freelancer
- plan out and take action on that new business you have always wanted
- actually write and send out your monthly newsletter
- find an accountability partner

Personal finances
- put away $100 per month towards a new car payment
- save $6,000 by the end of the year towards that new house
- pay off your credit card by December 31st
- consolidate your finances and get a line of credit in place by April

Business finances
- ask for a raise on your next anniversary or review date
- work part time to save extra for that house down payment
- pick up one new client for your freelance business each month
- invest $1,000 into the stock market
- replace 50% of your salary by working on your own business
- quit your job by December 31st and work from home
- look for a new higher paying position and secure it by the end of the year

Goals related to improving your skills
- finish your degree by June
- become a licensed instructor
- offer to teach a class at your gym
- learn a foreign language
- take a cooking class
- take a computer class

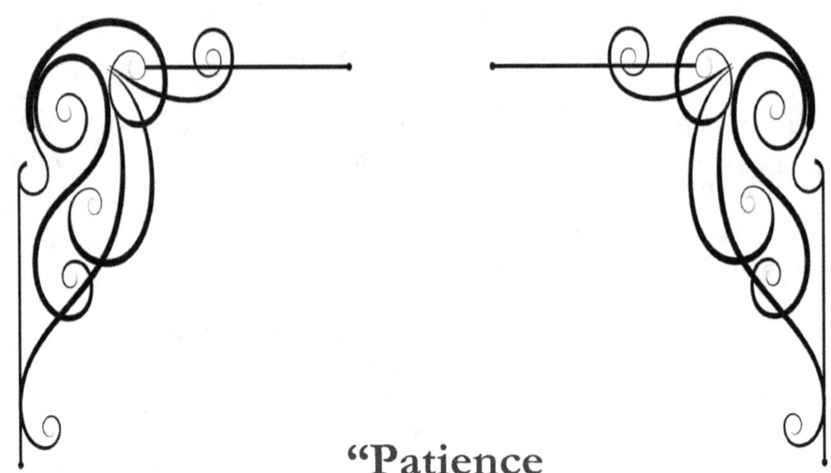

"**Patience**
is not passive waiting.
Patience
is active acceptance of the
process required to attain your
goals and dreams."

~ Ray Davis

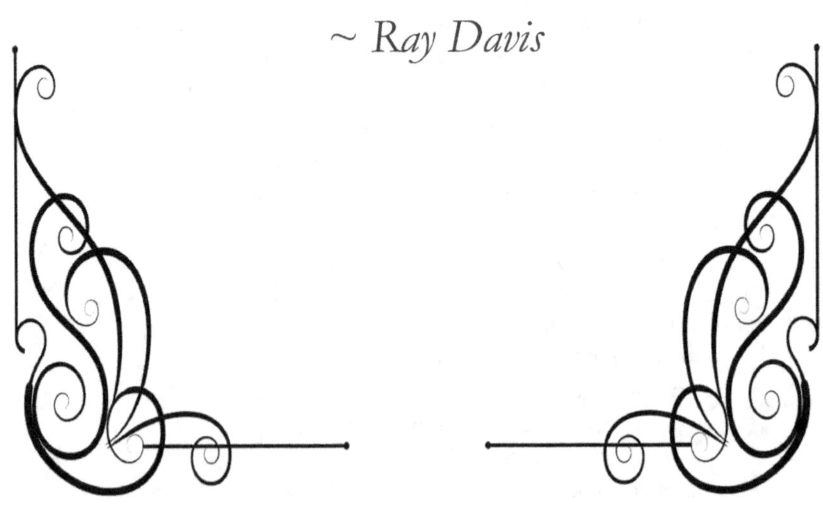

Health and fitness related goals

- lose 10 pounds by April
- train for a 5k and enter one in July
- fit into those tight-fitting jeans by the end of summer
- fit into that bathing suit by June
- cut out one can of soda per day
- reduce the amount of coffee you drink by one cup per day
- eat 100 calories fewer every day
- take a 15 minute walk every day
- get up and do 50 sit ups each morning before getting dressed
- lose 2 inches of your waist by august
- lose 52 pounds by December 31st
- compete in a 10k by the end of the year
- learn how to ride a bike, play golf etc.
- taking swimming or dancing lessons
- take self-defense classes
- cut out sugar in your diet by reducing the amount you use in your coffee and tea
- use sea salt
- buy organic fruits and vegetables
- stick to meatless Mondays for the entire year
- only order take out and fast foods once per month

Dating and relationship goals

- plan a trip for your wedding anniversary this year
- schedule a date night at least once a week
- celebrate Valentine's day
- write your loved one a love letter and mail it to them
- make a break from your relationship by April 1st
- send that someone special flowers
- tell your partner you love them once a week at least
- hug your partner every day
- start going out on dates again
- join that dating site by February 1st
- take a getaway weekend to celebrate a long weekend

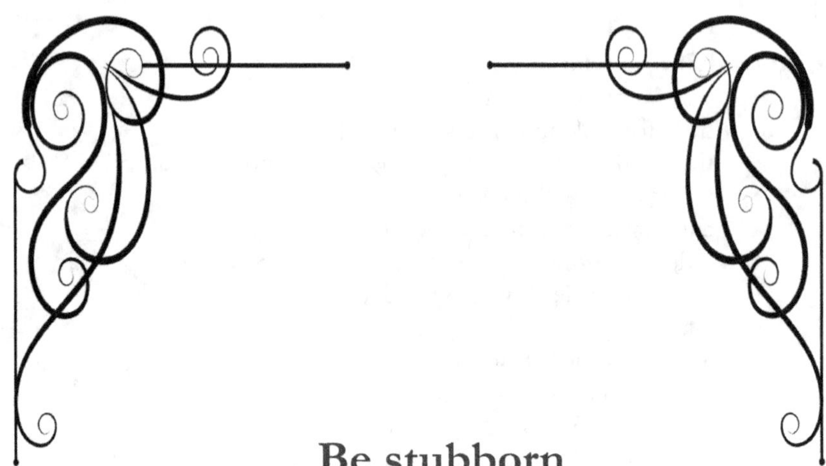

**Be stubborn
about your goals,
and flexible about your
methods.**

**You will face many defeats
in your life,
but never let yourself be
defeated.**

~ Maya Angelou

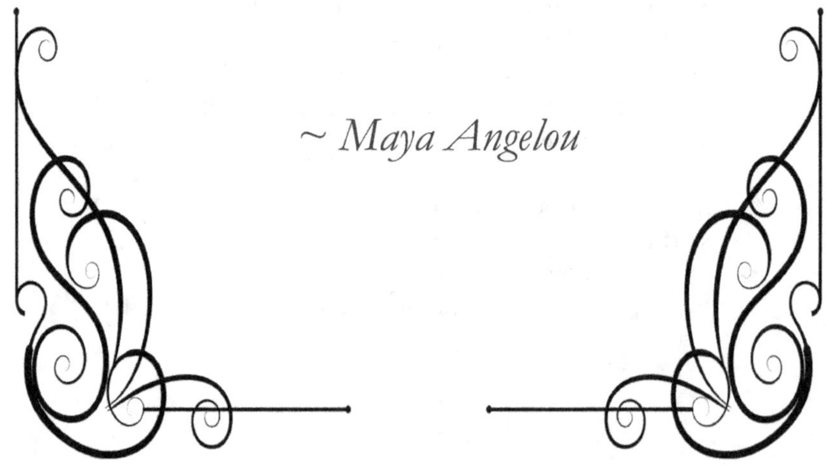

Family related goals
- read your young kids a bedtime story
- watch a movie at least once a week with your kids
- dedicate Sunday's as family time for the entire summer
- take your kids to the golf course with you
- put the kids into swimming lessons
- visit your own parents at least once a month
- take your family to see a sports game at least once
- enjoy a family night out at the movies
- book a family camping trip
- buy that new puppy your promised by spring
- help your parents move closer to you
- hold that garage sale in May
- plan a family BBQ for the July long weekend
- take your kids to see a wildlife safari
- see a wild animal in its natural habit
- go on a boat ride

Travel and dream related goals
- go skiing with your family
- visit Disney World before your youngest goes to school
- buy or rent an RV for your summer vacation
- visit local tourist attractions
- plan to drive across the country this summer
- visit your dream destination
- drive to the nearest ocean and walk on the beach
- go to a professional sports game this year
- finish writing that book you started by November
- go on a European river cruise in the spring
- buy that vacation home you have always wanted
- send the kids to their grandparents for the month of august
- teach your son/daughter to drive this summer
- drive a sports car
- plan out your trip to Australia by August
- visit the great wall of China
- visit your birth town and take your family with you

Use any of the above goals as suggestions to match your own dreams and desires. Remember that you can achieve great things in all areas of your live. You just need the determination to take action and stick to it.

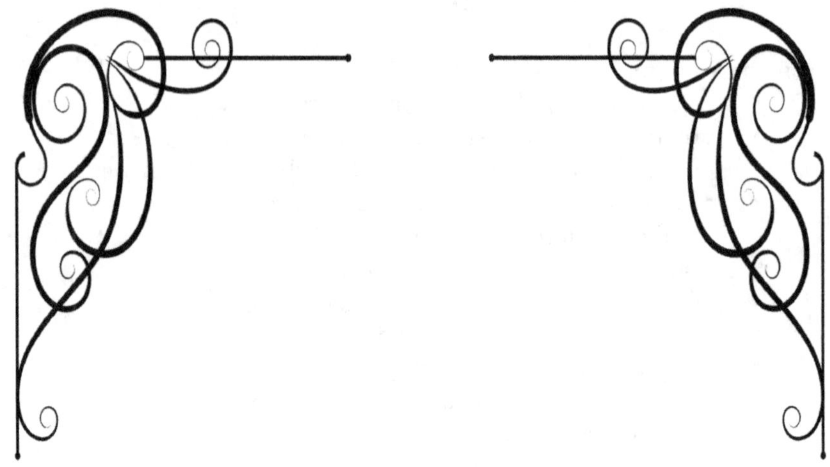

"The greatest amount of
wasted time is the time not
getting started."

~ *Dawson Trotman*

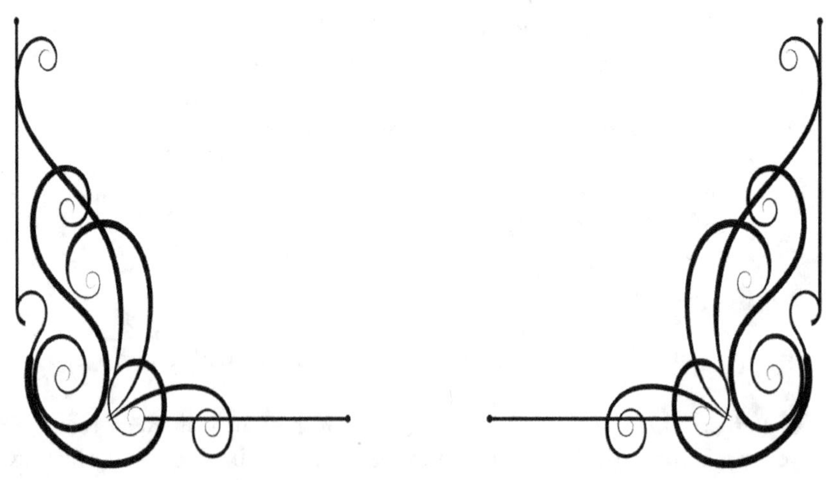

CONCLUSION

Start now, make this the year you turn your resolution into a personal revolution.

If you take only one thing away from this book, please let it be this:

The traditional New Year's Resolution needs to be treated like a goal that is written down with specific, measurable action steps and due dates.

It sounds pretty simple, but just doing that will significantly increase the likelihood that you stick to your New Year's resolution. Making your steps along the way doable and fun will drastically improve your success.

Setting a goal doesn't mean you will reach it, but you will succeed more often than not if you set it according to the information in this book and then commit to following the goal setting tips described.

Now when the clocks strike midnight on New Year's you'll be prepared to make a resolution that sticks.

All the best to you, and Happy New Year!

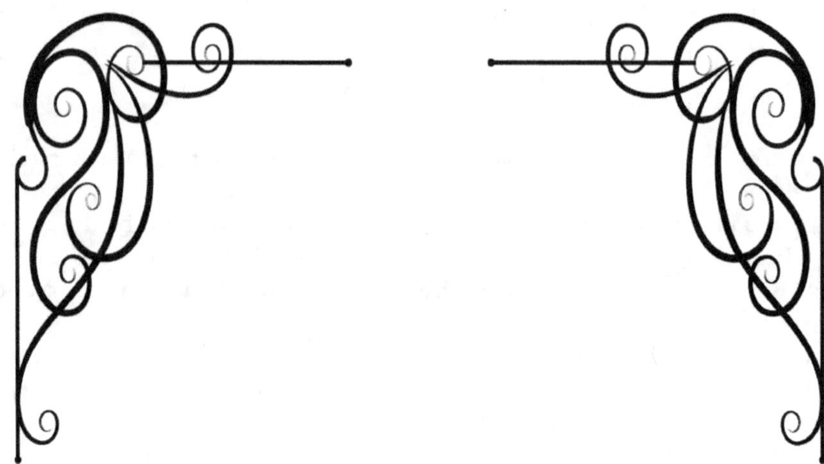

"The object of a New Year
is not that
we should have
a new year.

It is that we should have
a new soul."

~G.K. Chesterton

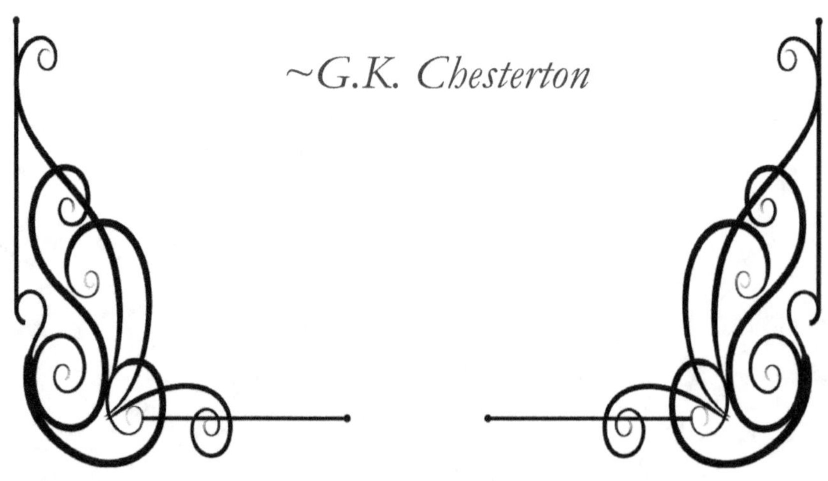

ABOUT THE AUTHOR

People often search for solutions during times of suffering. Carol has firsthand experience seeking solutions for the suffering of her patients, her clients and herself. Hope is always her first step in healing suffering. Hope helps you begin again, dream for a different tomorrow and start taking action today.

Carol Stockall is a caregiver who has worn many hats. She began as a candy-striper, and later became a nurse, doctor, coach and counselor. A lifelong learner, Carol has a host of academic and professional letters behind her name including; BA, RN, MD, FRCPC, ACC, MC, and CCC. With decades of professional health care experience combined with a lifetime of personal experience Carol has earned a "PhD in life" that only comes with experience.

Today Carol's most known for her work coaching and counseling caregivers. She is a professional coach, certified by Erickson Coaching International, the International Coach Federation and the Physician Coaching Institute. Carol holds a post-degree diploma in Interprofessional Mental Health and a Master's degree in Counseling. Her thesis work was focused on burnout with a special interest in mindfulness to build balance and restore resilience.

Carol is dedicated to helping people achieve their goals and live their best life. Get Carol's **FREE WEEKLY PLANNER** – MAKE YOUR RESOLUTION A REALITY to help you track your resolve and keep your resolution. Download it now at:

http://carolstockall.com/make-your-resolution-a-reality

The most conscientious caregivers often make caring for someone else a priority while they sacrifice their own self-care. It's easy for the life goals of the caregiver to get lost along the way. Carol helps caregivers fulfill their own goals while making life-balance and self-care a priority. Carol offers coaching, counseling and a variety of resources for caregivers seeking self-fulfillment.

For a **FREE COACHING SESSION** – MAKE YOUR RESOLUTION A REALITY contact Carol now at:

http://carolstockall.com/complimentary-coaching-session.

To connect with Carol, visit her at www.CarolStockall.com.